RAND

Evaluating the Feasibility of Developing National Outcomes Data Bases to Assist Patients with Making Treatment Decisions

Cheryl L. Damberg, Liisa Hiatt, Kitty S. Chan, Rebecca Nolind, Michael Greenberg, Michael Steinberg, Matthias Schonlau, Jennifer Malin, and Elizabeth A. McGlynn

Prepared for the
Agency for Healthcare Research and Quality

RAND Health

The research described in this report was sponsored by the Agency for Healthcare Research and Quality. The research was conducted within RAND Health.

Library of Congress Cataloging-in-Publication Data

Evaluating the feasibility of developing national outcomes databases to assist patients with making treatment decisions / Cheryl L. Damberg ... [et al.].
    p. cm.
    "MR-1708."
    Includes bibliographical references.
    ISBN 0-8330-3420-0 (pbk.)
    1. Outcome assessment (Medical care)—Databases—United States. 2. Patients—Decision making—Databases—United States. 3. Patient education—Databases—United States.
    [DNLM: 1. Databases—United States. 2. Treatment Outcome—United States. 3. Decision Making—United States. 4. Patient Participation—United States. W 84 AA1 E83 2003] I. Damberg, Cheryl. II. Rand Corporation.

R853.087E95 2003
362.1'0285—dc21

                                                                        2003008618

A profile of RAND Health, abstracts of its publications, and ordering information can be found on the RAND Health home page at www.rand.org/health.

RAND is a nonprofit institution that helps improve policy and decisionmaking through research and analysis. RAND® is a registered trademark. RAND's publications do not necessarily reflect the opinions or policies of its research sponsors.

Published 2003 by RAND
1700 Main Street, P.O. Box 2138, Santa Monica, CA 90407-2138
1200 South Hayes Street, Arlington, VA 22202-5050
201 North Craig Street, Suite 202, Pittsburgh, PA 15213-1516
RAND URL: http://www.rand.org/
To order RAND documents or to obtain additional information, contact Distribution Services: Telephone: (310) 451-7002; Fax: (310) 451-6915; Email: order@rand.org

PREFACE

This report examines the potential for, and range of issues associated with, establishing national health outcomes data bases to help patients and their physicians evaluate tradeoffs among various treatment options. Patients are frequently faced with more than one treatment option and often those treatments have multiple outcomes that need to be understood and evaluated in terms of their risks and benefits to the patient. This work builds on previous Agency for Healthcare Research and Quality (AHRQ) - sponsored expert meetings funded by the Kanter Family Foundation—which focused on the possibility of developing data systems that would allow patients to share information with other patients about the decisions they had made when confronted with alternative treatment choices and the outcomes they had experienced.

The study is based on a formal review of the shared decision-making literature as it relates to creating decision support tools for patients; on interviews and consultative discussions with patient and physician representatives; and on a review of existing data collection efforts to establish what is feasible, what are the inherent challenges, and what are the lessons from these efforts that could guide the development of national outcomes data bases. This report should be of particular interest to government agencies and professional organizations whose responsibilities include the collection and analysis of data regarding the outcomes of treatment, and the dissemination and use of those results by patients and their physicians.

CONTENTS

TABLES

EXECUTIVE SUMMARY

Background

At some point in our lives, each of us will need medical care to treat an acute or chronic health condition. As patients, we frequently face difficult treatment decisions, needing to assess tradeoffs between various treatment options—such as whether to "do nothing" (i.e., watchful waiting), choose medication therapy, or have surgery. Patients increasingly are being encouraged to become more active participants in their care, including making decisions about treatment choices. However, for patients to be able to weigh tradeoffs and participate in decisions about their care, they must have access to information on the consequences or outcomes of different treatments. Information on the consequences or outcomes of various treatment options is generally not available to support informed decision-making by patients and their physicians.

Clinical trials often do not assess and compare the efficacy of various treatments for the same medical condition. And where clinical-trial data do exist, it is frequently difficult to use the results to help patients understand the outcomes they might actually experience. The reasons include the homogeneity of patients enrolled in clinical trials, the lack of consistent outcome measures, the failure to focus on outcomes of interest to patients, and results derived from interventions that do not reflect current or actual practice in most settings. When "outcomes" information is available, it usually is not readily accessible to patients, in a format that is easily understood, or tailored to address the unique needs of patients like themselves—namely, to address the question, what happens to "People Like Me" who choose this treatment?

The purpose of this research was to provide the Agency for Healthcare Research and Quality (AHRQ) with information that would contribute to an understanding of the need for and feasibility of establishing operational national outcomes data bases that could be used by patients and providers to make more informed treatment decisions. The "People Like Me" concept involves capturing longitudinal outcomes information on a wide range of patients undergoing various treatments for a select clinical condition. This information would then be packaged and made available for use by patients and physicians to understand what happens to People Like Me who choose a particular treatment and/or to compare treatments.

Study Objectives

This report summarizes the findings of RAND's assessment of the need for and issues related to the feasibility of establishing two separate outcomes data bases—one for prostate cancer and another for surgical treatment for patients with osteoarthritis. The two conditions were selected to illustrate the range of challenges and opportunities that would be encountered in establishing national outcomes data bases for various clinical conditions.

The study focused on the following:

- Examining the need for outcomes data bases, as determined by a review of the research literature on shared decision-making and through structured discussions with patients who have the clinical condition and physicians who treat those patients
- Defining the set of questions patients and doctors want answered
- Identifying existing data bases that collect longitudinal outcomes data on patients who have the two conditions
- Assessing whether existing data bases address, either partly or fully, the questions of interest, and whether they provide a ready platform for use by patients and physicians in a People Like Me context
- Examining the lessons learned from those who have developed outcomes data bases, such as exploring recruitment of patients and physicians, selection bias, development and maintenance issues, and costs
- Defining key parameters that should be addressed in constructing the data base (e.g., number of patients required, how the data need to be stratified to answer questions more closely tailored to specific patients)
- Defining next steps and recommendations for AHRQ regarding the development of patient-centered national outcomes data bases.

Findings

Based on our review of prostate cancer and osteoarthritis as two conditions that illustrate the complexity of treatment choices faced by patients, we found a very strong desire among patients to have access to an information source that would not only explain what their condition is but would also help them understand what the various treatment options are and what outcomes (i.e., survival, functioning, side effects) people like themselves could expect from each of the various treatment options. Overwhelmingly, patients observed that information was difficult to obtain, was not synthesized and presented in a way to allow them to understand the trade-offs, and rarely offered insights as to what their own experience might be given their unique characteristics (e.g., age, race/ethnicity, gender, health status, stage of disease). Patients with prostate cancer and osteoarthritis also described relying heavily on other patients for information in the absence of information that was presented from the patient's perspective as to what they might experience—as well as on the Internet, where they acknowledged it was difficult to assess the accuracy of the information presented.

Perhaps because of their own difficulties in finding information, patients indicated they would be very willing to participate in a longitudinal outcomes data base, particularly if they understood that it would benefit future patients in their quest for information. While patients wanted to ensure that their own personal data were protected, they did not see privacy issues as an obstacle to their participation. Patients expressed a preference for the federal government—such as the National Institutes of Health—or a nationally respected and trusted organization (e.g., American Cancer Society) to operate such a system because those groups would have no vested interest in any particular form of treatment and were more likely to present accurate information. Patients noted they would have reservations about participating if the project were sponsored and operated by a pharmaceutical company or medical device manufacturer that produces a treatment. Those firms might be less willing to provide objective information and/or might try to market products directly to patients participating in the data base project.

Providers also expressed considerable support for the People Like Me data base concept, particularly as it pertained to obtaining information on the clinical benefit of various therapies for different types of patients. They also seemed interested in finding ways to better organize and present information to help patients understand treatment options because they currently struggle with how best to communicate with patients given a wide range of patient preferences for information—from "you make the decision, doctor" to "I want to know all my choices and what is going to happen as a result of each choice." Both providers and patients agreed that a national outcomes data base would provide an important tool for shared decision-making between patients and providers, something that is currently lacking.

Providers did express concern about the validity of the data base depending on how the sample of patients whose data make up the data base were chosen. They underscored the complexity of gaining representative participation by providers and patients in a voluntary data base that reflected a sample of patients with the condition—which could potentially lead to a biased sample. Physicians expressed some reservations about patients being able to view the outcomes information by themselves outside of the doctor-patient consultation; however, they acknowledged that the Internet has greatly transformed the discussions that doctors have with their patients, so that patients often come to the doctor armed with information they want to discuss. Physicians' primary concern regarding the construction of the data base seemed to be with the accuracy and validity of the information in the system.

With respect to the feasibility of developing national outcomes data bases, it was clear from our research that efforts have already been made—both in the United States and abroad—to develop data collection systems that longitudinally track patient outcomes. Outside the United States, these more frequently consist of disease registries that capture 100 percent of the patients with a particular condition or treatment—typically within national health systems. The information derived from the longitudinal data base systems that we reviewed was viewed as extremely valuable for research purposes to understand how patients fare under different forms of treatment—especially as treatments evolve after the clinical trial stage. While not yet fully realizing their potential in this regard, the data bases were seen as a valuable tool to support clinicians in their interactions with patients. None of the projects that we reviewed had taken the next step of making the information available for direct use by patients, although the developers noted that this was an important audience for the information, and they were interested in finding ways to translate existing data for use by consumers and exploring how they might modify their data base efforts in the future to support greater shared decision-making between physicians and patients.

The existing longitudinal data base efforts demonstrate that establishing an outcomes data base is technically feasible and is valued by end users, but that substantial resources are required to design and operate them. The amount of resources required largely depends on the number of patients and providers who participate in the data base to produce statistically reliable results by different profiles of interest to patients (how many People Like Me demographic and clinical characteristics are accounted for), the amount of data required to be captured (how many data elements), the frequency and intensity of follow up efforts to track patients over time, the scope of the effort (how many conditions and interventions are being monitored), and the investment made to translate and present the results in a way that patients can understand and use to make informed choices. To establish and operate a national outcomes data base, the investment is likely to range from $5 to $25 million annually—with the costs determined by the factors noted above.

It is clear from our work that there is keen interest among patients to have a People Like Me resource, that providers support this activity, and that smaller-scale efforts have been successfully designed and implemented. Prior to undertaking the establishment of a national outcomes data base for any medical condition, we recommend conducting meetings with patient and provider representatives to solicit their support for and input into the design of the system. While various health conditions share similar features, we did identify through the patient-provider discussions some unique factors across different conditions that would affect the design and implementation of the data base. The patient and provider meetings will be an essential step to firmly define the scope of the project, the goals of the data base, how data will be captured (which outcomes are of interest and how are they measured), how the data are analyzed, and how and what data will be shared with patients and providers.

ACKNOWLEDGMENTS

Funding for this work was provided under contract (HHS 282-00-005-TO5) from the Agency for Healthcare Research and Quality, US Department of Health and Human Services. In conducting this work, we very much appreciated the thoughtful guidance, feedback, and support of our project officer, Dr. Carolyn Clancy.

We wish to acknowledge and thank the patient and provider representatives who participated in our consultative meetings and provided ongoing input and feedback as we explored the range of issues associated with developing patient outcomes data bases. Additionally, we are grateful for the careful and thoughtful review of our work by Dr. Judith Hibbard and Dr. John Wennberg, who provided important contributions to the final report.

We are indebted to the contributions made by Landon Donsbach, who helped the research team organize the consultative meetings, locate research materials, and produce the final report. Lastly, our thanks to Miriam Polon for her editorial assistance.

CHAPTER 1:
INTRODUCTION

Problem Statement

Patients who are diagnosed with a particular medical condition frequently must choose among treatments that will minimize pain, reduce disability, and/or enhance their likelihood of survival. When information is not available on the outcomes of many treatments, patients cannot evaluate the trade-offs among the options. Patients are particularly interested in how people fare who are similar to them based on clinical characteristics (e.g., for prostate cancer the PSA value, Gleason Score, presence of other comorbid conditions) or demographic characteristics (e.g., gender, age, race/ethnicity). Information that does exist on the outcomes of care is often not well organized or easily accessible and interpretable to patients. Rarely, if ever, is the information tailored to the characteristics of an individual patient.

In addition, there are gaps in the outcomes information that hinder patients' and health professionals' ability to predict the consequences of treatment and the trade-offs between different treatment options. For example, one type of treatment for a condition may have undergone rigorous evaluation (e.g., randomized clinical trial) while the other treatments may have had no thorough review to evaluate their benefits and risks. Randomized controlled clinical trials (RCTs) are expensive and complex undertakings, and a substantial number of medical treatments never have received this level of evaluation. Although RCTs are the gold standard for determining whether a treatment is efficacious, they do not provide information regarding the effectiveness of treatment (i.e., what outcomes are achieved when the average patient sees the average physician). Until recently, clinical trials focused only on clinical endpoints such as survival, ignoring other outcomes of keen interest to patients (e.g., quality-of-life, daily functioning).

Clinical trial results are limited in their utility for helping patients make individual treatment choices. Clinical trials typically compare a specific treatment versus doing nothing, rather than comparing two different treatment alternatives. Clinical trials also tend to enroll a homogenous population of patients who are not representative of the broader population of patients with the condition. For example, a new medication may only be tested in a clinical trial on white males with no other comorbid conditions. Once we know the effect of the treatment for this narrow population of white, otherwise healthy males, the question is, does the medication exhibit the same effects in women and/or persons of color and for those with comorbities (e.g., high blood pressure, diabetes)? Having information routinely collected on a large number of average people treated with the range of alternative treatments would allow continual examination of whether it is reasonable to assume that non-studied populations are likely to experience the same benefits of treatment as observed for patients in the controlled studies.

The Food and Drug Administration (FDA), which has regulatory oversight for drugs and medical devices, reviews the evidence from clinical trials and approves drugs deemed safe and efficacious. Once approved, the drugs and devices are nearly always applied in a much broader population of patients than were included in the clinical trials. Problems with drugs or devices that do not get identified during the clinical trial stage often are revealed through post-marketing surveillance when the treatment is applied to a much larger and more diverse patient population. During the post-marketing surveillance stage, problems with a device or drug are identified and reported by patients and their doctors—although there is no systematic longitudinal tracking system for all treatments to facilitate better understanding of the differential impact of treatments on different types of patients. No federal regulatory structure provides oversight on the safety or efficacy of surgery unless the surgical treatment involves the use of a device. Again, the development of longitudinal data bases that track the safety and effectiveness of various treatments would be of considerable use to patients who seek to understand whether a given treatment option has benefit for them and what side effects or complications they might experience by selecting a particular treatment course.

Another problem with research information derived from clinical trials—which capture an intervention at a specific point in time—is that it may not accurately reflect current medical practice. Technological changes, which may occur once the therapy is applied in general practice, can improve patients' outcomes. Changes in the formulation or dosing of drugs may reduce side effects. Use of technologies in the hands of less-skilled providers can result in outcomes being worse. Research studies are frozen at the point in time they were conducted, and their findings may not generalize once the treatment is applied broadly in the population and evolves in response to the experience gained from widespread use. An outcomes data base could provide up-to-date information on current experiences of persons undergoing different treatment options.

Outcomes research has added significantly to our understanding about how the choices among treatments affect patients' experiences in everyday life. The tools used to evaluate patient outcomes increasingly are being used in clinical research studies and by doctors in everyday practice. Unfortunately, we lack this type of information on more-established therapies that came into use before studies started incorporating the new measures. Moreover, the relevant information is not readily accessible when tough decisions have to be made. Further, even in the newer studies, different surveys may be used, which may make it difficult or impossible to compare the results of different treatments. For example, a recent review identified nine different quality-of-life surveys that are used in studies of men with prostate cancer (Sommers and Ramsey, 1999). They found that the surveys covered different domains of health and emphasized different outcome dimensions; additionally, that no one survey had been applied to all treatments or used with men across the age spectrum with different stages of cancer. So, even physicians dedicated to giving their patients the best information on what to expect from one treatment versus another would not be able to assemble comparable information. Standardizing the information routinely collected about people undergoing treatment for a disease would substantially improve the ability of patients and physicians to make decisions about treatment options.

Helping Patients Make the Right Treatment Choices for Themselves

Patients want and need information that allows them to understand the consequences of initiating treatment for a particular clinical condition and also to weigh tradeoffs between different treatments when options exist—so that they can make the right treatment choice given their circumstances and preferences. In the future, patients will be increasingly challenged to select among alternative treatment options given the growth in federal investment in the National Institutes of Health for conducting research to identify new and better treatments across a broad array of medical conditions.

The field of outcomes research has underscored a critical point about medical management and decision-making: For many clinical conditions, there is no single treatment or approach that is appropriate for every patient. Rather, there are many situations in which the medical outcomes for alternative treatment approaches are comparable but involve different tradeoffs in terms of risks, recovery time, and individual preferences for expected side effects of treatment. As Wennberg and colleagues (1993) observe, "when the outcomes of a particular treatment are multiple and when more than one treatment option exists, an optimal treatment choice for individuals depends on the evaluations they give to the risks and benefits associated with the outcomes that matter to them." Patients require outcomes information to help them evaluate risks and benefits associated with alternative treatments—however, this type of information is rarely available, organized, and presented in a way that patients can understand and use to inform their choice of treatment.

In 1989, the Agency for Health Care Policy and Research (AHCPR) funded the Patient Outcomes Research Teams (PORTs) to attempt to answer questions about the effectiveness and cost-effectiveness of available treatments for common clinical conditions (e.g., back pain, acute myocardial infarction, diabetes, prostate disease). The PORTs were to address the following questions: what works and at what cost; for which patients or subgroups of patients; when; why is there variation in the use of treatments, and what can be done to reduce variation (Freund et al., 1999). The PORTs were to use readily available data—observational in nature—to advance our understanding of outcomes of care as applied to patients in everyday practice. The PORT approach stood in contrast to the traditional approach of conducting randomized clinical trials (RCTs) to answer questions regarding whether one treatment is more effective than another. The use of observational rather than experimental data to advance our understanding of differences in patient outcomes from medical care, however, was not without controversy.

Peto and Baigent (1998) expressed concern regarding the limitations of using observational data for outcomes assessment, stating that the strength of RCTs rests in their ability to avoid the confounding that is associated with unmeasured initial differences among treatment cohorts. Randomization is designed to produce patient groups that are truly comparable with respect to known and unknown prognostic factors at baseline, whereas observational studies run the risk of not controlling for unrecognized confounding factors that may bias the results. Yet, a review by Benson and Hartz (2000), designed to compare differences between observational studies and RCTs, found little evidence that estimates of treatment effects in observational trials reported after 1984 were consistently larger than, or qualitatively different from, those obtained in RCTs.

Wennberg et al. (1993) countered that RCTs also have the potential for confounding, including a bias that occurs from failure to investigate the interdependency of therapeutic effects with patient preferences, placebo, and compliance. Not much is known about the capacity of RCTs to establish accurate outcome probabilities because the estimates obtained under randomization may not predict outcomes under open choice. It is not known whether patient preferences influence the effectiveness of treatments or outcomes—something that RCTs do not control for (McPherson et al., 1997). These researchers noted that probabilities for symptom reduction and other outcomes estimates produced under traditional RCTs (i.e., patients randomly assigned a treatment) versus an alternative study design, the Preference Clinical Trial or PCT (i.e., patients choose among all treatments after being offered information about risk and benefits of conventional and experimental treatments) decision-making would likely not be the same. They hypothesized that expectations associated with active patient choice should result in better outcomes for all treatments. The PCT is more observational in its approach to evaluating outcomes—allowing patients to understand tradeoffs associated with all of the various treatment options, letting them choose the treatment, and then following what happens to people who choose different treatments. Wennberg and his colleagues emphasized that researchers must identify all of the outcomes that matter to patients and then be able to estimate accurately the probabilities that the various outcomes will occur, given the treatment used and conditioned on patients' comorbidities and severity of illness. The proposed People Like Me approach to identifying the outcomes of interest to patients and building data bases that help provide this information could focus attention on which clinical trials to fund and which outcomes would need to be derived from longitudinal tracking of patients in an observational data base.

To help patients understand the consequences of treatment, a variety of efforts have been undertaken to develop and evaluate new approaches to involve patients in making treatment decisions and self-management of their chronic illnesses. We reviewed the literature on shared decision-making in the context of this project, with the specific goal of eliciting key considerations that might affect the design of patient-centered outcomes data bases (see Chapter 3). Shared decision-making tools remain largely a "research" activity, and they have not been widely or systematically adopted in the routine practice of medicine. Consumers are seeking out information to guide their decisions, much of it from the Internet (Berland et al., 2001) and from patient support groups that try to fill the needs of other patients like themselves. However, the locus of most efforts of consumers to inform themselves and share health information with others is peripheral to the physician-patient encounter, thus creating the potential for individuals to receive conflicting information from clinicians and other sources.

At the same time that patients are tapping into new and diverse sources of health information, many new evidence-based tools designed to inform clinicians and improve decision-making have emerged and been absorbed into practice (e.g., Partin nomograms for prostate cancer treatment). However, there is not yet a strategy that combines the use of data to inform decisions made by patients and clinicians in a way that is both relevant to patients' experiences and preferences and clinically credible.

How to Fill the Information Gap

In 2000, AHRQ sponsored two expert meetings funded by the Kanter Family Foundation. The meetings focused on a discussion of the potential utility of developing data systems that would allow patients to share information with other patients about the decisions they had made when confronted with alternative treatment choices and the outcomes they experienced. In conceptualizing the data base, it was thought that combining the experiences of many patients could help them contribute to the development of an accurate picture of what happens to people like themselves, without compromising their own privacy. Moreover, it would promote the development of evidence-based tools and data systems to help clinicians and patients make informed decisions when faced with a similar array of valid choices.

From these meetings, the expert participants underscored that for any condition or disease, development of a system would require

- a data base of information from a large number of individuals with a given condition to permit analyses within demographic or other subcategories relevant to experiencing different outcomes (e.g., stage of disease, functional status)
- an effective user interface that would assist physicians and patients obtain answers to questions in real time.

One strategy for filling the information gaps is to develop national longitudinal outcomes data bases or registries that could be used to produce information for patients and their physicians to use in making treatment decisions. The information derived from such data bases would also help fill the information gap regarding where quality-of-care problems exist and identify opportunities for improving the safety and quality of care delivered to patients across the United States.

To generate information on outcomes from various treatments for a clinical condition, it would be necessary to collect a range of information, including immutable patient demographic characteristics, baseline prognostic factors, treatments the patient receives, and subsequent outcomes over many years from patients diagnosed with that condition. This is a considerable challenge both in terms of logistics and costs, and may be an appropriate strategy for certain clinical conditions. Recognizing that developing an outcomes data base may not be an appropriate strategy in many cases (because of feasibility and cost considerations), we start by defining a set of criteria that can be used as an initial screen to determine whether a given clinical condition is a suitable candidate for this type of investment (see Chapter 2).

Assessing the Need for and Feasibility of Establishing National Outcomes Data Bases

To understand what would be involved in establishing patient-centered outcomes data bases that could be used by patients and physicians, AHRQ contracted with RAND to assess the need for and feasibility of establishing outcomes data bases, using two clinical conditions as models, to explore the range of issues that need to be considered—size, scope, participation by patients and physicians, and cost. For the two conditions selected for review, the feasibility assessment would

- specify a framework to guide the development of data bases across a variety of diseases
- explore the need for creating outcomes data bases for two model conditions
- assess the readiness for implementation for the two model conditions
- evaluate the willingness of patients and providers to participate in a national outcomes data base and identify potential barriers to participation that would need to be addressed for the data base to succeed
- evaluate the feasibility and costs associated with initial development and ongoing maintenance of the two model data bases.

Specifically, RAND was asked to identify factors that could facilitate or impede the ongoing data collection in the process of routine patient care. This report summarizes the findings from our assessment.

The organization of the report reflects the major tasks that RAND was asked to perform. Because not all conditions may be suitable for creating a national outcomes data base, Chapter 2 presents a framework for selecting clinical conditions and describes the process used to conduct the assessment. For the purpose of this study, two conditions were selected to make concrete the challenges and opportunities that would be encountered in establishing national outcomes data bases for various clinical conditions. Chapter 3 contains a review of the literature on shared decision-making and, drawing from this work, highlights key design considerations for establishing national outcomes data bases. Chapter 4 provides a detailed assessment of the need for and feasibility of establishing a prostate cancer outcomes data base. Chapter 5 is dedicated to a similar assessment for osteoarthritis. Chapter 6 summarizes key factors that we have identified that must be considered and addressed to establish outcomes data bases, defines next steps, and makes recommendations regarding the development of patient-centered national outcomes data bases.

CHAPTER 2:
A FRAMEWORK FOR ASSESSING THE FEASIBILITY OF ESTABLISHING NATIONAL OUTCOMES DATA BASES

The design and construction of a national outcomes data base is a substantial undertaking, financially and logistically, and one that may not be appropriate for all clinical conditions. It is therefore important to establish a set of criteria that can be used to help guide decisions about whether a condition is a worthy candidate for such a data base. These criteria can be used as a first-level screen for assessing the likelihood for success of making an investment in data collection that will require long-term participation by a large number of patients and clinicians. Moreover, it is important to examine the nature and extent of existing data collection efforts for the condition of interest, and to determine whether they can be used to produce the information of interest; if they provide a foundation to build on or if a de novo effort is required; and what lessons can be gleaned from the experiences of these prior efforts to collect longitudinal data on the patient and clinical population of interest.

In conducting the assessment, RAND applied a framework that comprised (1) articulating the purpose of a national outcomes data base and defining the ways in which such data can be useful for patients and providers; (2) establishing a set of criteria for selecting candidate clinical conditions; (3) drawing from the shared decision-making literature to guide the construction of a patient-centered national outcomes data bases (see Chapter 3); and reviewing existing data bases (see Chapters 4 and 5).

Purpose of a National Outcomes Data Base

The purpose of creating the proposed People Like Me outcomes data bases is to provide information about experience with a course or courses of treatment, tailored to those demographic and clinical characteristics of patients that are known to influence the outcomes, and to help patients and their physicians make treatment decisions that lead to the best outcomes given patient preferences. This process can occur by making information readily available about the experience of different courses of treatment—whether drawn from clinical trials, treatment registries, or surveys—stratified by key patient characteristics. Depending on the condition selected, the way in which the outcomes data base is built may differ (i.e., a newly created registry versus combining existing data bases from clinical and observational studies); however, the basic data base concept being proposed is observational, following a cohort of patients who have faced a treatment decision and chosen (or had chosen for them) one of several available treatments (including watchful waiting). Once the information is gathered and organized, the information then must be presented in formats that can assist patients and clinicians with understanding the state of knowledge regarding different treatment courses for the selected health conditions and patient experiences with those treatments.

Criteria for Selecting Conditions for Review

The project team, in collaboration with the AHRQ project leader, selected eight candidate clinical conditions for initial evaluation with the objective of narrowing the clinical set to two conditions. The two chosen clinical conditions would serve as models to explore and contrast a range of issues that would influence the feasibility of establishing national outcomes data bases. We purposely selected two conditions that would have different design implications to illustrate the range of issues associated with such a project (e.g., existence or lack of existence of data bases, evidence-based treatment guidelines versus consensus based guidelines, content). An assessment of all possible clinical conditions for potential investment in creating outcomes data bases was outside the scope of this project.

The eight conditions selected for consideration were arthritis, breast cancer, congestive heart failure, epilepsy, infertility, multiple sclerosis, Parkinson's disease, and prostate cancer. Each of these conditions was evaluated against the following criteria, which were developed to be used as an initial screen for determining whether a given clinical condition was a good candidate for a data base.

Selection Criteria

1. *Prevalence of the condition in the population.* The condition should affect a large number of people to ensure a large enough pool of potential participants and to maximize the use of the data base and their effect on treatment decisions. A larger pool of patients will also facilitate subgroup analyses.

2. *Significant impact on health.* The condition should significantly affect the person's health and functioning (i.e., mortality, morbidity, and quality-of-life).

3. *Existence of treatment alternatives.* The treatment course should involve clear treatment decision points or alternative actions that patients could take (e.g., medical versus surgical interventions, watchful waiting versus active intervention)—so that the availability of information would help

patients evaluate and make more-informed treatment decisions with their clinicians.

4. *Variation in treatment experiences*. Although the treatment alternatives may have comparable long-term outcomes (e.g., mortality), differences should exist in the experience (i.e., process, intermediate outcomes) a patient will have. These differences should represent key determinants of patient choices.

5. *Existing data collection efforts*. The existence of a national data base that tracks selected aspects of care, which might serve as a foundation for building a more robust data base to assist with decision-making.

6. *Treatment alternatives that imply different cost profiles*. The different treatment alternatives have different costs and patients face varying out-of-pocket expenditures for care.

7. *Subgroup differences in outcomes*. The conditions are characterized by differences or disparities in treatment patterns for subgroups of the population (subgroups could be defined by demographic and/or clinical characteristics).

8. *An evolving knowledge base*. The conditions should reflect areas where the science of treatment is evolving or changing, so that there is a lack of information on the effectiveness of treatment alternatives (i.e., randomized controlled trials).

9. *Willingness of patients and providers to participate*. A high likelihood exists that clinicians and patients would be willing to participate in supplying information to create the data base.

In addition to these criteria, in our consultative discussions with patients and clinicians, three additional criteria were identified as important factors that would make a condition a good candidate for data base development: (1) A highly mobilized and vocal patient constituency exists that can advocate for the creation of the data base and that can mobilize patients to participate in the effort; (2) The condition is life-threatening or debilitating; and (3) The treatment is ongoing (or potentially recurrent) rather than a single occurrence.

Condition Selection Overview

To select two conditions for the People Like Me feasibility assessment, we applied the criteria listed above to eight candidate conditions: arthritis, congestive heart failure, epilepsy, infertility, multiple sclerosis, Parkinson's disease, prostate cancer, and breast cancer. Below, we briefly summarize our findings for each condition. In consultation with AHRQ, we decided a priori to examine one cancer condition and one non-cancer condition. We therefore organize our discussion by cancer and non-cancer conditions.

Non-Cancer Conditions

Arthritis. The Centers for Disease Control and Prevention (CDC) estimates that about 43 million Americans, or one out of every six individuals, have some form of arthritis. Furthermore, this number is expected to reach 60 million by the year 2020. In 1999, more than 17 percent of all disability among people over the age of 18 was caused by arthritis (Centers for Disease Control and Prevention, 2001). Osteoarthritis affects about 21 million people, making it the most common form of arthritis (Centers for Disease Control and Prevention, 2001). Arthritis is the leading cause of disability in the United States, and the daily activities of about 7 million Americans are limited by the disease. Arthritis, in all of its various forms, is responsible for 44 million outpatient visits and 750,000 hospitalizations each year. The annual medical cost of treating arthritis is $15 billion, and lost productivity accounts for an additional $50 billion annually in indirect economic costs (Centers for Disease Control and Prevention, 2001).

Depending on the severity of the pain and limitations in movement, patients usually have several different treatments from which to choose. Some patients may find it effective to use only one treatment, while others may need to combine several treatments to relieve pain and increase movement. Physical therapy, exercise, and Transcutaneous Electrical Nerve Stimulation (TENS) have been shown to be effective in reducing pain and increasing the ability to walk (Easton, 2001). Acetaminophen, NSAIDs, and COX-2 inhibitors have all been used successfully in treating osteoarthritis (Easton, 2001). When the pain is extreme or the range of motion is extremely limited, some patients may consider surgery for their osteoarthritis. Hip or knee replacement surgeries are treatment options when less invasive treatments fail. However, both are major surgeries that are expensive and can be dangerous to undergo (Easton, 2001).

While a number of the medications used to treat osteoarthritis have been studied in randomized controlled trials, the various treatments have never been compared against one another (i.e., medication versus surgery) and combination treatments have not been studied. Given a wide variety of available treatments and the lack of comparative information on the outcomes of these various treatments, it can be very difficult for patients to choose a treatment best suited for their circumstances.

Congestive Heart Failure. About 4.8 million Americans suffer from congestive heart failure (CHF), and about 400,000 new cases develop each year. In 1993, there were 42,000 deaths directly related to CHF (a four-fold increase from 1968) as well as another

219,000 deaths that were indirectly related to the disease. CHF is the most prevalent diagnosis among hospitalized patients over the age of 65: Approximately 20 percent of hospitalized patients in this age group have CHF as either a primary or secondary diagnosis. Between 1980 and 1993, the number of physicians' office visits for the condition increased by 70 percent. As the elderly population grows in size, these numbers are expected to increase (National Heart, Lung, and Blood Institute [NHLBI] Fact Sheet, 1996).

In 1993, the annual direct medical costs of treating congestive heart failure were estimated at $17.8 billion. This figure includes hospitalizations, doctor visits, home care, nursing home care, and medications; however, it does not take into account indirect costs attributable to the condition such as lost wages for caregivers or the emotional toll that the disease can have on a family (NHLBI Fact Sheet, 1996).

Many decisions need to be made in treating CHF, especially given new, experimental and very costly treatments that continue to be developed. Decisions about CHF treatment are frequently made by the doctors in emergency situations with little input from the patients. Many of the treatments are backed by data from multiple randomized control trials (i.e., the use of ACE inhibitors, beta-blockers, digitalis, etc.). In other cases, there is evidence from a single RCT or consensus on the part of physicians (i.e., use of calcium channel blocking drugs, routine use of nutritional supplements) (Gomberg-Maitland et al., 2001). The American College of Cardiology (ACC) and the American Heart Association (AHA) revised their guidelines concerning the evaluation and management of CHF in 2001 (American College of Cardiology and American Heart Association, 2001). The ACC and AHA guidelines do provide treatment guidance for subgroups of the population, including groups defined by gender, race, age, and comorbidities. A People Like Me data base could help clinicians and patients grapple with decisions about the array of new treatments.

Because a number of treatments are available to patients with CHF, including many that are still experimental, an outcomes data base could provide an opportunity to track and compare outcomes. However, because treatment decisions often have to be made immediately in an emergency or urgent situation, it is unclear whether patients would be able to use the information effectively to influence their course of treatment.

Epilepsy. Epilepsy is a syndrome of susceptibility to repeated seizures. Nearly 1.4 million people in the United States have epilepsy and most are under the age of 45 (Epilepsy, 1996). The prevalence of epilepsy is higher for African-Americans than whites in every age group except those ages 15 - 24. For persons ages 35 - 44, the prevalence among African-Americans is about 13 per 1,000 compared to four per 1,000 for whites. For persons ages 45 - 55, the prevalence among African-Americans is 10 per 1,000 persons compared to four per 1,000 for whites. The disease is also slightly more prevalent among women than men with 5.1 cases per 1,000 women compared to 4.2 cases per 1,000 men (Morbidity and Mortality Weekly Report, 1994). The incidence of epilepsy is 30 to 56 new cases per 100,000 persons annually (American College of Radiology, 1999).

Based on information from the Epilepsy Foundation of America (Epilepsy Foundation of America website, 2002), the annual costs approximate $12.5 billion in direct medical costs for all types of treatment and indirect costs resulting from lost wages. Between 20 and 30 percent of epileptic patients are unemployed because their condition prevents them from keeping a job. Many new, effective, and costly medications have become available for treatment in recent years, and medication can cost patients thousands of dollars a year. In addition to drug therapy, treatments are available for recalcitrant cases—these treatments include vagus nerve stimulation, which generally costs about $15,000, and neurosurgery, which is even more expensive.

The recommended initial treatment once a diagnosis of epilepsy has been made is the standard dose of a first-line antiepileptic drug. A number of randomized controlled trials have been conducted that demonstrate the effectiveness of certain drugs for different types of seizures, thus providing evidence-based guidance for making treatment decisions (Browne and Holmes, 2001). If the medicine does not control the seizures, causes too many side effects, or is too toxic, then the dosage may need to be adjusted. If the dosage cannot be increased enough to control the seizures without causing unacceptable toxicity, then a new medication will need to be prescribed. Patients and physicians may consider discontinuing anti-epileptic drugs under certain circumstances when the patient is seizure free. The probability of recurrent seizures once medication is discontinued is between 25 and 50 percent (Browne and Holmes, 2001). Vagus nerve stimulation is a procedure whereby an electrode is attached to the left vagus nerve and a generator is implanted in the chest wall. Regular pulses of electricity prevent or interrupt seizures. Brain surgery to remove the area of the brain that causes the seizures or interrupts the nerve pathways along which the seizure impulse travels is also an option (Benbadis and Tatum, 2001).

Although epilepsy affects a significant number of people and can have a profound impact on the lives of the people it affects, with appropriate clinical management it can usually be controlled to the point that the person can live a normal life. In many cases, the person can discontinue the medications entirely after a few years.

Infertility. Infertility is generally defined as the inability to conceive after a year of intercourse without the use of birth control. In 1995, 15 percent of all women of reproductive age (15 - 44 years), or about 9.3 million women, reported ever receiving infertility services, and about 6.7 million of them (10 percent of women of reproductive age) were found to have infertility problems. Infertility rates vary widely by age group. About four percent of women ages 15 - 24 had infertility problems compared with 13 percent of women ages 25 - 34 and 21 percent of women ages 35 to 44 (Mosher and Bachrach, 1996). The population with fertility problems is very similar to the general population in terms of race and socioeconomic status. Infertility problems disproportionately affect older women of childbearing age (Stephen and Chandra, 2000).

In 1984 dollars, a successful pregnancy achieved through any form of infertility treatment cost an average of $10,700. However, the costs of treating infertility vary greatly depending on the underlying cause of the infertility and the treatment necessary (Cooper, 1986). A 1996 study found similar costs for the insurance company (about $10,500) in addition to about 35 percent more in patient cost-sharing for diagnosis and simple treatments. More-complex procedures such as in vitro or other assisted reproductive techniques were not included (Bates and Bates, 1996).

If it is possible to define the cause of infertility, then treatment will depend on the reason for infertility. If the problem is with the male, then intrauterine insemination or intracytoplasmic sperm injection are usually attempted. If the woman is not ovulating, then drugs are used to attempt to induce ovulation and intrauterine insemination can still be tried. If this does not work, there are other ovulation-inducing therapies as well. If ovulation is confirmed and semen analysis is normal, then the couple may try the drug therapy combined with intrauterine insemination anyway. If none of these therapies are successful, diagnostic testing with laproscopy is usually continued. If everything looks normal, these procedures are usually attempted again. However, if the fallopian tubes are blocked, the treatment may be a surgical attempt to open the blocked tube or to begin assisted reproductive techniques (Battacharya and Hall, 2000).

Infertility is an important health problem affecting approximately 10 percent of couples of reproductive age. It has a significant effect on quality-of-life including sexual problems, marital problems, depression, and potential financial hardship if treatments are pursued. There are clear patient-centered issues regarding complex treatment decisions for infertility, such as whether to be treated versus whether to adopt a child, which make it a good candidate for shared decision-making and patient-physician discussion.

Multiple Sclerosis. Nationwide, there are approximately 250,000 to 350,000 cases of multiple sclerosis (MS). The prevalence of multiple sclerosis is between 57 and 140 per 100,000 and geography is a key factor in the observed variation in prevalence rates. The observed prevalence of MS is higher (110 to 140 per 100,000) among the population in areas above the 37th parallel, which runs from Newport News, VA, to Santa Cruz, CA, compared to areas below the 37th parallel (57 - 78 per 100,000). MS is more common among Caucasians, especially those of northern European descent. It is practically non-existent in the Inuit population, however. It affects two to three times as many women as men (National Multiple Sclerosis Society, 2001).

In 1994 dollars, the cost per person per year for treating multiple sclerosis was about $34,000 (Whetten-Goldstein et al., 1998). Annual direct and indirect costs for treating multiple sclerosis in the United States are estimated at $6.8 billion, and the lifetime cost of treating one person with multiple sclerosis can be as high as $2.2 million. These costs include personal health services, paid or unpaid care from professionals or relatives and friends, retraining, equipment, and earnings loss. There is also the emotional cost of dealing with the disease, since it often prevents the person from working and there is a high likelihood that a person with MS will be in a wheelchair (Whetten-Goldstein et al., 1998).

Many MS patients show signs of recovery without treatment after a relapse, though most clinicians recommend treating each episode. Clinicians have successfully used corticosteroids to shorten relapses and speed recovery, even though there is no strong evidence that they aid in long-term recovery (Polman and Uitdehaag, 2000). Eventually, relapsing/remitting multiple sclerosis develops into a secondary progressive stage, in which the attacks are less pronounced and the remissions occur less often. Interferon beta is the usual course of treatment for this phase as well (Polman and Uitdehaag, 2000).

The impact of multiple sclerosis on quality-of-life for those who suffer from it is severe. Most persons with the disease will be forced to quit their job after only one year and will find themselves in a wheelchair within 15 years. In addition, the costs per patient may be as high as several million dollars over the course of a lifetime, placing a large burden both on health insurance companies and the patients and their families. However, there are few treatment options and most of the treatments are through drug therapy. Given limited choices of therapy and the fact that the disease affects many fewer people than the other conditions evaluated for study, MS would rank lower among the various conditions as a good candidate for a People Like Me data base.

Parkinson's Disease. The estimated number of people with Parkinson's disease in the United States is between 500,000 and 1,500,000. Based on information from the Mayo Clinic, the prevalence of Parkinson's is about 200 cases per 100,000 people and the incidence of new cases is about 20 per 100,000 per year. The average age of onset of Parkinson's is 60, although about 5 percent of cases occur before the age of 40 and are classified as early-onset Parkinson's. While there is some indication that the prevalence of the disease is lower among Africans, Japanese, and Chinese, it is unclear whether this translates into lower prevalence among African-Americans, Japanese-Americans, and Chinese-Americans. There also seems to be a slightly higher prevalence among men than women, since six in 10 cases are male (Koller, 1993).

According to the Parkinson's Action Network, the annual cost of drug therapy for early-stage Parkinson's is about $2,000 - $7,000. For more advanced stages of the disease, the costs can run much higher. Treatment for Parkinson's-related falls, which occur in about 38 percent of those with Parkinson's, can be up to $40,000 or more, including hospitalization. In addition, about 30 percent of those with Parkinson's will lose their jobs within a year, so disability subsidies can be as much as $30,000 annually. With progressive Parkinson's, the patient often requires assisted living and nursing home care, which can cost more than $100,000 per patient (Parkinson's Action Network, 1999).

Parkinson's results from a severe shortage of dopamine, a substance that allows people to move normally. The main treatment for Parkinson's is pharmacological, but there are several classes of drugs that can be used in treatment of the disease. In addition to these basic treatments, physicians will usually treat some of the symptoms of Parkinson's, such as the tremors normally associated with the disease. While the ideal treatment would slow the progression of Parkinson's, the main treatment goals are often to relieve the symptoms, so that they do not interfere with the patient's daily life, and to reduce the chances of complications (Young, 1999). Surgery is considered a last resort, and is utilized only when the patient fails to respond to pharmacological treatment and does not have any cardiopulmonary risk factors for surgery. Several different surgeries may be appropriate for treating Parkinson's (Young, 1999).

Parkinson's disease affects a large number of people and significantly affects quality-of-life. As the disease progresses, it can lead to the need for assisted living, which can be very difficult and costly. Although there are some choices in treatment, the main treatment is pharmacological. Surgery is used only as a last resort. Therefore, patients have few decision-making options. While the costs of treating the disease are high, they are less than those of osteoarthritis and prostate cancer.

Cancer Conditions

Breast Cancer. Approximately 192,000 new cases and 40,000 deaths from breast cancer occur annually in the United States. Breast cancer is the leading cancer diagnosis among women and ranks second after lung cancer for all deaths from cancer among women. Overall, American women have a one-in-eight lifetime chance of being diagnosed with breast cancer. However, the probability of this diagnosis increases with age. A woman between 30 and 40 has a one-in-257 chance of being diagnosed with breast cancer as compared to a one-in-24 chance for a woman between 70 and 80 (National Institutes of Health, 2001).

The American Cancer Society estimates that expenditures for breast cancer treatment in the United States are about $6 billion annually in direct medical costs. The cost of breast cancer treatment is significantly lower when it is detected early. A 1996 study estimates that treating breast cancer in a preinvasive stage costs $30,000 to $40,000 less compared to treating it in a later invasive stage (Legorreta et al., 1996).

With a diagnosis of lobular carcinoma in situ (LCIS-stage 0), the preferred treatment is observation, since LCIS is not considered cancer but a risk factor. For stage I or II breast cancer (primary tumors less than 5 cm), a number of randomized clinical trials have shown that mastectomy or lumpectomy followed by radiation treatment is clinically medically equivalent with regard to outcomes. For women whose breast cancer is metastatic, hormonal therapy is indicated if her hormone receptors are estrogen- and/or progesterone-positive. If not, chemotherapy will often be of benefit (National Comprehensive Cancer Network, 2000).

Prevalence, cost of treatment and impact on quality-of-life are all significant for breast cancer. Treatments for breast cancer have generally been well evaluated in clinical trials. In addition, at most stages of treatment, clear evidence-based guidelines exist on the course of treatment, and there is very little controversy over what works, except at very late stages when the cancer has metastasized. However, at various points in the treatment course, patients may be asked to make a choice about treatment that may involve different side effects, duration, and difficulty of treatment. The main choice a woman given a diagnosis of breast cancer may be faced with is whether to undergo a lumpectomy with subsequent radiotherapy or a mastectomy, where the radiotherapy is probably not indicated. These two choices have been shown to have clinically equivalent outcomes. Most of the other treatment choices (i.e., tamoxifen versus chemotherapy) have more to do with what will work for the woman's particular clinical profile. It is also important to note that breast cancer patients are highly interested in complementary and alternative medicines, none of which has been rigorously evaluated to guide treatment decisions.

Prostate Cancer. Prostate cancer is the most common cancer diagnosis and is second only to lung cancer in cancer-related deaths among American men. The American Cancer Society projects that in 2002, 189,000 new cases of prostate cancer will be diagnosed (American Cancer Society website, 2002). In 2000, there were roughly 32,000 deaths attributable to prostate cancer. Approximately 70 percent of all cases are diagnosed in men age 65 years and older. Prostate cancer is about twice as common in African-American men as in white men.

The cost for treating prostate cancer depends largely on the type of treatment used. A 2000 study of over 10,000 men treated for early-stage prostate cancer found that the average costs of the initial work up for diagnosis, treatment, and six-month follow up ranged from $12,000 to $30,300, depending on the type of treatment (Brandeis et al., 2000). Treating with radical prostatectomy and adjuvant radiation is the most expensive, with an average cost of $30,300. Radical prostatectomy alone had a mean cost of $18,300, and the adjuvant radiation alone typically had costs of $15,100. The least expensive form of treatment for early-stage prostate cancer was brachytherapy (radiation through radioactive seeds implanted directly in the tumor), at about $12,000 (Brandeis et al., 2000). Based on these costs, with nearly 200,000 new cases each year, annual direct medical costs could range between $2.4 and $6 million. All of the above costs are for treating early-stages of prostate cancer. When the cancer is discovered in later stages, it is likely to be much more expensive since extended treatments may be necessary. For metastatic disease, costs could include extended rounds of hormone treatments, chemotherapy, and palliative care, which could lead to even higher treatment costs.

For localized and regional disease, the most common treatments are radical prostatectomy or radiation therapy, although some physicians may recommend "watchful waiting" or hormone therapy depending on patient characteristics (such as age). Once the cancer has metastasized, there is no longer a choice in treatments. At this point, androgen ablation, either with hormone treatment or through orchiectomy, is the recommended treatment. If the androgen ablation ceases to contain the disease, then chemotherapy is used as a treatment of last resort (Pienta et al., 2001).

The prostate-specific antigen (PSA) screening test is now widely used, and an increasing share of prostate cancers are being detected at earlier stages where men have more options for treatment. At most stages of the disease, at least two treatment choices may be equally effective in terms of long-term outcomes but may have markedly different intermediate outcomes on sexual, urinary, and bowel functioning. In contrast to breast cancer, for which there have been multiple randomized controlled trials to compare alternative treatment therapies, studies to compare the benefits of various treatment options for prostate cancer are almost entirely lacking. The exception is a recent study that randomly assigned newly diagnosed prostate cancer patients to watchful waiting versus radical prostatectomy and compared patients in the two groups on mortality, metastasis-free survival, and local progression (Holmberg et al., 2002). This study found no significant difference between surgery and watchful waiting in terms of overall survival, while radical prostatectomy significantly reduced disease-specific mortality.

Prostate cancer represented an excellent candidate for exploring the range of issues associated with creating an outcomes data base because of the size of the population affected, the fact that prostate cancer can result in death, that there are treatment choices with varying consequences for the patient, and that little or no information is available to compare these choices.

Conclusions

Each of these clinical conditions meets many or all of the selection criteria enumerated above. For the purposes of this study, however, we were requested to narrow the list to two conditions as a means to explore the range of issues related to creating People Like Me outcomes data bases. Based on our review of the eight candidate conditions against the selection criteria, RAND, in consultation with AHRQ, selected prostate cancer and osteoarthritis as the conditions to use to examine the feasibility of establishing outcomes data bases for use by patients and providers.

These two conditions are very different in terms of the types of treatment choices and the consequences of those choices on the health and functioning of the patient, as well as the costs to the patient. Prostate cancer results in significant mortality among men, and while osteoarthritis is not a life-threatening situation it can cause severe disability over a person's lifetime. Data bases exist for prostate cancer, (e.g., SEER, CaPSURE, PCOS) which may offer potential platforms on which to build a larger data base, although they are currently not structured to produce and make available information for use by patients. Some arthritis data bases exist, but they do not focus on osteoarthritis (the subset we selected for study), and most look at medications rather than surgical treatments. With respect to osteoarthritis, there has been a proliferation of surgical procedures and some of them are perceived to be underused.

Both prostate cancer and osteoarthritis have several treatment options that require patients and their doctors to make complex decisions. Additionally, once diagnosed with the condition, patients have time to engage in shared-process for both conditions. Few of the treatments for either condition have undergone randomized controlled trials to compare differences in outcomes (intermediate or long-term), so there is need for additional information on outcomes that patients are likely to experience. For both conditions, there are disparities in outcomes for subgroups of the population. Prostate cancer is about twice as common in African-American men as in white men. Arthritis is more common among women, older people, those in rural areas and those with low education or income levels. Both diseases present challenges for establishing an outcomes data base; however, there is ample opportunity to expand our understanding of the effects of different courses of treatment for two medical conditions that have little existing comparative outcomes information.

Process for Conducting the Feasibility Assessment

Once the two model conditions were selected, the project team did the following:

1. Identified examples of existing longitudinal data bases as well as data tools that were being used with patients to help them understand treatment outcomes.

2. Interviewed project staff within each of the identified data bases to examine what information they were collecting, how the data were used, and what the issues were in developing and maintaining a longitudinal data base to track patient outcomes.

3. Identified a list of physician leaders and patient advocates in each clinical area who could speak to the problems of existing information on which to base treatment decisions.

4. Held meetings with the physician and patient advocate leaders to reflect on the need for a People Like Me data base, articulate the questions the data base should be designed to answer, and explore the range of issues and challenges in collecting data.

5. Summarized the information from these discussions, interviews, and reviews of existing data collection efforts to guide future work on developing national outcomes data bases tailored to address the questions of People Like Me.

Chapters 4 (prostate cancer) and 5 (osteoarthritis) describe the work and findings from the feasibility assessment. Another important step in our assessment process was an examination of the literature on shared decision-making (Chapter 3) to identify issues that have implications for using a People Like Me outcomes data base to provide decision support tools for patients and physicians.

CHAPTER 3:
SHARED DECISION-MAKING: A REVIEW OF THE LITERATURE

Introduction

Shared decision-making has gained greater relevance for clinical medicine in recent years. When treatment alternatives are available but none is clearly superior, there is greater recognition that patient values and preferences should factor into decision-making (Barry, 1999). However, incorporating shared decision-making into clinical practice has been challenging, owing to: (1) the lack of role models and training for clinicians; (2) the limited time available during clinical encounters; (3) the complexity of evaluating and clearly communicating to patients the tradeoffs in the risks and benefits of treatment; and (4) the lack of good, relevant data to inform decision-making (Dunn et al., 2001; Braddock et al., 1999; Barry, 1999).

Shared decision-making programs and decision aids offer an opportunity to address some of these problems by providing information and decision assistance to patients outside the clinical encounter. While their specific goals and content vary, these aids generally aim to inform patients about likely outcomes of therapeutic options, incorporate patient values in weighing the benefits and risks of treatment, and encourage patient participation in care decisions. Evaluations of these programs suggest that they can increase patient knowledge, reduce decisional conflict, influence patient behavior, and affect treatment choice (Hersey et al., 1997; O'Connor et al., 2003). However, the reliance of many decision aids on using clinical trial data for their probabilities of therapeutic risks and benefits (Murray et al., 2001a, 2001b; O'Connor et al., 1999) raises several concerns. First, the currency of the data used in the decision aid will determine their utility for informing treatment decision-making, especially for conditions in which available treatments change rapidly. Second, if the study intervals for trials used to calculate probabilities in the decision aid are not sufficiently long, the long-term consequences of treatment exposure and complications may not be well described. Finally, the stringent eligibility criteria imposed by most randomized clinical trials may make their results less applicable for patients who do not fit their eligibility profile (e.g., patients with multiple health problems or those who take a number of different medications). Many developers have responded to these concerns by adopting update policies for their products (O'Connor et al., 1999; O'Connor et al., 2003). In addition, a transparent evidence base can help users gauge the usefulness and generalizability of a particular decision aid. However, a lag time is still likely to exist between when new data, whether for new treatments or from new studies, become available and when they are incorporated in updates. Data banks or data bases may offer an alternative strategy for treatment decision support by providing a dynamic stream of data on the therapeutic experiences of a broad range of patients and serving as a repository of outcomes for existing and novel therapies.

However, experience with the use of data bases for this purpose is limited, and an assessment of the market for these outcomes data bases, potential implementation strategies, and the practical issues associated with incorporating their use within the flow of clinical care—including facilitators and barriers—is necessary before additional steps can be taken to develop them for decision support. To identify user and design issues that should be considered when evaluating the feasibility of developing a data base to assist patients in treatment decision-making, we reviewed the literature to identify the characteristics of patients who are most likely to participate in shared decision-making, what information patients want and what format they want it in, and the likelihood of physician support for these data bases. We also reviewed the evidence on the use and effectiveness of shared decision-making programs and decision aids for informing patient decision-making.

The State of Patient Involvement in Clinical Decision-Making

For many patients, their physicians are the primary source of information about treatment options. However, evidence to date suggests that the degree of information-sharing and collaborative decision-making in clinical practice is often quite low. For example, when presented with hypothetical patients with no significant medical history and normal physical examinations, most physicians participating in a study of clinical decision-making indicated that their decision to order mammograms or prostate-specific antigen (PSA) tests was independent of patient preference (Dunn et al., 2001). In fact, one-third of the participants would not discuss cancer screening with the patients at all. These physician attitudes are confirmed by the experience of real patients. In a study of preferred and perceived decision-making roles in 233 cancer patients, 45 percent preferred a shared role, but only 24 percent felt that decision-making was shared. In addition, patients who perceived their role as being more passive than they would have liked indicated that they wanted more information on treatment options and their side effects, a chance to voice their concerns, and greater reassurance that they would be well looked after (Gattellari et al., 2001).

In an effort to critically evaluate the quality of information-sharing during the clinical encounter, Braddock et al. (1999) analyzed audiotapes from 1,057 patient-physician encounters for elements of informed decision-making, using preestablished criteria. The authors found that only 9 percent of decisions met the definition of completeness for informed decision-making. Even when the least stringent definition was applied, only 20 percent of discussions were considered complete. Basic decisions were most often completely informed (17 percent), but few intermediate or complex decisions were (less than 1 percent), despite the fact that intermediate and complex decisions made up nearly half of the decisions observed. Across the three levels of decision complexity, the nature of the decision was discussed most frequently (66-84 percent). Treatment alternatives (6 - 30 percent), pros and cons (2 - 26 percent), or uncertainties associated with the decision (1 - 17 percent) were rarely discussed. Physicians sometimes discussed patients' role in decision-making (5 - 18 percent) and elicited patients' preferences (18 - 27 percent), but rarely explored whether patients understood the decision (1 - 7 percent).

Lack of time was cited as one reason physicians limit patient involvement in decision-making (Dunn et al., 2001). Indeed, Braddock et al. (1999) found that during visits averaging between 14 and 17 minutes, about two to three patient concerns were addressed. However, physicians do include more elements of informed decision-making for complex decisions (Braddock et al., 1999). Other factors, such as language barriers, may offer partial explanations for why some decisions were poorly informed (Dunn et al., 2001). Overall, these results raise concerns regarding whether patients are adequately involved in clinical decision-making. However, these studies are cross-sectional, and it is possible that many patient concerns had already been addressed in prior visits or that resources (e.g., nurse practitioners, health educators, and decision aids) providing necessary information for informed decision-making were available to patients outside the clinical encounter.

Patients' Need for Information
The Level of Patient Information Need

While the degree of information-sharing during the clinical encounter appears limited, patients consistently report a high demand for information. Strull et al. (1984) reported that 41 percent of 210 patients with hypertension wanted more information about their condition. Similarly, Kennelly and Bowling (2001) found, in focus groups with 38 cardiac patients (aged 56 and older), that participants did not feel they received sufficient information from their doctors to make informed choices.

Patients and their families appear to fill some of the information gap by accessing health websites on the Internet. A report on the use of online health resources, funded by the Pew Charitable Trusts, estimated that 52 million Americans, or 55 percent of those with Internet access, used the Web to get health or medical information (Fox and Rainie, 2000). Of those who sought health information for themselves, 47 percent indicated that the material they found influenced decisions made about treatment or care. However, the quality (i.e., accuracy and completeness) of the information on these websites is not monitored, and a recent study reported that coverage of important clinical information has been poor (Berland et al., 2001). For example, the authors reported an average of 16 percent, 20 percent, 27 percent, and 35 percent of key questions about breast cancer, depression, childhood asthma, and obesity, respectively, received no coverage at English-language sites and 49 percent, 61 percent, 33 percent, and 69 percent of the elements for these four conditions received no coverage at Spanish-language sites. Despite these quality concerns, however, the popularity of Internet health resources reflects the strong demand patients and their families have for readily available information about clinical conditions and treatment options.

What Kinds of Information do Patients Look For?

Fox and Rainie (2000) found that among those using online health resources, 70 percent reported that their last online search was for a specific condition. Of those who looked for medical information for a specific condition, 48 percent looked for information on symptoms, 30 percent sought information about treatments or medicines, and 29 percent looked for information on what happens to people who contract a specific illness. Kennelly and Bowling (2001) found that participants in their focus groups wanted more information about their condition as well as balanced information about treatment options and their associated health outcomes. Similarly, Gattellari et al. (2001) found that cancer patients wanted feedback on the progression of their disease, information about their prognoses, and the risks and benefits associated with different treatment options and side effects.

Patient Preferences for a Decision-Making Role

While the demand for information was uniformly high, the level of involvement patients desire in decision-making is less predictable (Robinson and Thomson, 2001). Studies have reported that a large proportion of patients want to participate in therapeutic decisions (69 percent of 439 interactions between hospitalized cancer patients and oncologists in Blanchard et al., 1988; 45 percent of 233 cancer patients in Gattellari et al., 2001). However, these studies also found a sizable minority who preferred to delegate responsibility for treatment decisions to physicians (31 percent in Blanchard et al., 1988; 37 percent in Gattellari et al., 2001). This variability in patient preferences for involvement has led researchers to search for factors that can predict the role patients want in treatment decision-making.

Demographic and Socioeconomic Effects on Decision-Making Preferences

A number of demographic and socioeconomic factors, including age, gender, and education, have been observed to influence patients' preferences for participation in treatment decision-making. In particular, younger age is associated with a desire for greater involvement. For example, Vertinsky et al. (1974) observed that the desire for participation decreased with age (Spearman $r = -0.23$, $p = 0.001$, $N = 200$, randomly sampled from the community). Similarly, Blanchard et al. (1988), Degner and Sloan (1992), and Deber et al. (1996) reported that younger cancer patients expressed a greater desire for an active role in decision-making and that being older was associated with a desire to delegate treatment decision responsibilities to physicians. However, it is possible that the observed association with age may be partially or primarily due to a cohort effect. Females were also more likely to desire an active role in decision-making, although the effect was less consistent. Vertinsky et al. (1974) reported that females were less likely to want to delegate decision-making responsibilities to physicians, and Blanchard et al. (1988) observed that female cancer patients were more likely to want an active role. However, McKinstry (2000), who studied 410 patients' preferences for a shared or directed approach in five hypothetical clinical scenarios, found no major association with gender. Degner and Sloan (1992) observed that a higher level of education was associated with a desire for greater responsibility for decision-making in a newly diagnosed cancer sample, and McKinstry (2000) found that higher social class was associated with a desire for a shared style of decision-making. Despite these effects, demographic and socioeconomic variables accounted for only a small proportion of the variance in decision-making preferences (15 percent in Degner and Sloan, 1992). Furthermore, the relationship between these variables and role preferences are likely to be complex, and neither Vertinsky et al. (1974) nor Degner and Sloan (1992) believed that these variables could adequately predict decision-making preferences in patients.

Health Status Effects on Decision-Making Preferences

Studies have found that patient preference for involvement declines as they move along the spectrum from wellness to illness. For example, Vertinsky et al. (1974) reported that greater frequency of visits to the physician ($r = -0.31$, $p = 0.001$) and longer hospitalizations ($r = -0.22$, $p = 0.003$) were associated with a lower desire for an active role in decision-making. Similarly, Degner and Sloan (1992) reported that 59 percent of 428 cancer patients, but only 9 percent of 271 subjects among the general public wanted a passive role in decision-making. The authors noted that recent diagnosis in the cancer patients might have contributed to their desire to delegate decision-making responsibility, while the hypothetical scenario posed to the public might have led these subjects to overestimate their desire for an active decision-making role. However, Blanchard et al. (1988) also found that patients with advanced disease and lower functional status were less likely to want involvement in decision-making. On the other hand, Degner and Sloan (1992) reported that neither symptom distress levels nor stage of disease (cancer) were associated with patient role preference in decision-making. In addition, 51 percent of cancer patients and 46 percent of the general public wanted their physician and family to share responsibility for decision-making if they were too ill to participate. Finally, Gattellari et al. (2001) reported that patients with metastatic cancer were twice as likely to perceive that their role was more passive than they would have liked (adjusted odds ratio: 2.01; 95% CI: 1.13, 3.59).

Despite evidence of demographic, socioeconomic, and health effects, the variability in decision-making preferences remains largely unexplained. It is important to note that the cross-sectional nature of this research makes it difficult to determine if different preference sets reflect types of patients or states of interest that may be influenced by experience or education. For example, it has been suggested that patients may be reluctant to participate in decision-making because they are overwhelmed by the amount of information, the complexity of different choices, and the anxiety associated with the need to make the "right" decision (Frosch and Kaplan, 1999), a reluctance that could be overcome by a well-designed decision support aid. Furthermore, a positive experience in collaborative decision-making or greater knowledge about their condition may lead patients to desire a more active role in the future. However, without adequate follow up, the nature of such effects is unknown. This issue has particular relevance for patients with chronic diseases who become increasingly knowledgeable about their illness and must make multiple decisions over time (Watt, 2000). Furthermore, preferences for decision-making roles may be influenced by factors, such as the dynamics of the patient-physician relationship, that can change over time or are amenable to change through patient and physician intervention (Guadagnoli and Ward, 1998).

Contextual Influences on Shared Decision-Making

Contextual factors, such as organizational structure and the nature of the patient-physician relationship, can affect the propensity of patients and physicians to engage in shared decision-making. As part of a study of shared decision-making in medication use, Stevenson et al. (2000) asked 20 general practitioners to identify factors that would hinder or facilitate shared decision-making. In these discussions, physicians' beliefs about their patients' ability to understand medical language and medical problems was identified as a barrier to patient participation in decision-making. However, the physicians in the study also believed that an organizational shift toward greater teamwork with other health care professionals would generate more opportunities for shared decision-making. The nature of the patient-physician relationship may also affect the likelihood of patient involvement in treatment decision-making. One recent study with asthma patients suggests that the longer the patients' relationship with their doctor, the more their doctor will involve them in decision-making (Adams et al., 2001). Although these studies suggest that contextual factors can influence whether shared decision-making takes place, few studies have explicitly examined the effect of these factors on patient involvement in treatment decision-making.

Shared Decision-Making Programs and Decision Aids

Use of Shared Decision-Making Programs

Decision aids and shared decision-making programs have been developed for a variety of conditions including cancer, hypertension, and HIV/AIDS (Hersey et al., 1997; O'Connor et al., 2003; Hing et al., 2000; Montgomery et al., 2000; Murray et al., 2001a; 2001b). However, their rates of use appear to vary substantially (Hersey et al., 1997). For example, the PC-based Comprehensive Health Enhancement Support System (CHESS), placed in the homes of breast cancer (N = 400, Gustafson et al., 1996) and HIV/AIDS (N = 116, Boberg et al., 1995) patients, was heavily used. The program offered patients the opportunity to communicate with and share personal stories with other patients, as well as the ability to ask questions, retrieve information, and obtain assistance in decision-making tasks. Seventy-five percent of breast cancer patients referred to the CHESS program utilized the system and all of the HIV/AIDS patients used some aspect of the program, with services associated with enhancing social support being the most popular. Hersey et al. (1997) suggested that the breadth of offerings provided by CHESS might be a major factor promoting its acceptance because lower rates of use were observed for programs with narrower offerings.

Ease of access may also be important in enhancing rates of use. One study reported that only 14 percent of patients with low back pain used a tool that required an additional visit (Kamas, 1995). Programs that are readily accessible in patients' homes, either on a personal computer (e.g., CHESS) or through the Internet, might produce the highest levels of use. Finally, active promotion of the shared decision-making tool at the organizational level is likely to be necessary for continued use of the tool by patients; the use of an interactive videodisc system on benign prostatic hyperplasia dropped from 41 percent to 13 percent when the tool was no longer promoted by the care system (Wagner et al., 1995).

Patient Attitudes and Knowledge

Despite variability in rates of use, evaluations of shared decision-making programs and decision aids suggest that these aids are viewed positively by patients and can influence treatment decisions and patient behavior. Frosch et al. (2001) found, in a cross-sectional study of shared decision-making interventions for PSA tests, that 70 percent of all participants (N = 176) felt "somewhat positive" or "very positive" about participating in shared decision-making interventions. A greater percentage of those in the intervention groups expressed a desire for shared decision-making than in the usual care group (discussion: 55 percent; video: 67 percent; discussion + video: 70 percent; usual care: 47 percent). Those in the intervention groups were much less likely to want their physician to be the primary or only decision-maker (discussion: 2 percent; video: 4 percent; discussion + video: 8 percent; usual care: 49 percent). O'Connor et al.'s (2003) systematic review also found patients were more likely to take an active role in decision-making (pooled relative risk = 1.83, 95% CI = 1.02, 3.27).

The literature on decision-making programs and decision aids also suggest that these aids can increase patient knowledge of their condition and its treatment. Hersey et al. (1997) found that in eight of nine randomized trials of interactive videodiscs, videotapes, or brochures/fact sheets, users of these aids reported greater knowledge. O'Connor et al. (2003) estimated in their systematic review that average knowledge scores improved 9 to 28 points out of 100 (weighted mean difference = 19, 95% CI = 13, 25) when decision aids were used compared with usual care. They also found that patients who received a detailed decision aid that included descriptions of probability estimates were more likely to have realistic expectations of treatment risks and benefits than those who were given usual care (pooled relative risk = 1.48, 95% CI = 1.3, 1.8).

Treatment Selection

The effects of decision aids on treatment selection were variable. O'Connor et al.'s (2003) systematic review did not find that decision aids affected patients' decisions to circumcise male newborns or to get genetic screening for breast cancer. However, a 76 percent increase in preference was observed for hepatitis B vaccine in one study (Clancy et al., 1988) and a 25 percent reduction in the use of warfarin was observed in another (Man-Son-Hing et al., 1999). The review also noted a nonsignificant trend, between 21 and 42 percent, toward reducing patient preference for invasive procedures in studies of patient preference for major surgery.

Although these results suggest that decision aids can sometimes influence treatment selection, it is unclear whether these aids actually help patients achieve better downstream effects, such as persistence with choice or fewer regrets with treatment decisions (O'Connor et al., 1999). One study found that a substantial proportion of men who were previously treated for metastatic prostate cancer (23 percent of 201) regretted their choice (Clark et al., 2001). However, the limited empirical data currently available suggests that decision aids can do little to improve these downstream outcomes (Goel, 2001; O'Connor et al., 2003).

Overall Effects of Decision Aids

In general, decision aids appear to make patients be more knowledgeable about treatment options and have more realistic expectations about the risks and benefits of different therapies. Furthermore, there is evidence to suggest that decision aids can encourage more active participation in treatment decision-making and lead to decisions that are more informed and consistent with patients' personal values. However, their utilization rate and effects on treatment selection have been variable, and limited evidence is available to indicate that decisions made after using these aids produce greater persistence with chosen therapy or reduce decisional regret. Furthermore, more research is needed on how patients' sociodemographic characteristics, literacy level, and personal predisposition affect the way they access, use, and benefit from decision aids (O'Connor et al., 2003).

Patient Perspectives on Risk Information: Content and Format

In What Format Do Patients Want the Information?

Health information may be perceived as more useful when it is tailored to the patient. Jones et al. (1999) conducted a randomized clinical trial of 525 cancer patients that compared the effect of health information tailored to a patient's medical record with general information. The authors found that two-thirds of subjects who were given access to both personalized and general health information chose the personalized system first. Those in the personalized system group were also more likely to be satisfied, to think that the information was relevant, and to feel that they had learned something new. Patients in the personalized information system group were also more likely to use the computer in the follow up visits (20/169 versus 4/155, $p = 0.002$). Finally, a systematic review by Edwards et al. (2000) indicated that individualized risk estimates produced stronger intervention effects, suggesting that probability estimates can be effective for improving outcomes, particularly if tailored to the individual.

Treatments often produce adverse events, which can range in severity from a mild rash to death. Relating the severity of these events and the likelihood they will take place is known as risk communication. Research on risk communication suggests that patients can find risk information difficult to understand, especially when expressed in numeric terms (Edwards and Elwyn, 2001; Kennelly and Bowling, 2001; Lloyd, 2001). These studies have also found that although some prefer quantitative presentation of risks, many prefer to reinterpret numeric risks presented qualitatively (e.g., high or low).

It is important to note that how the information is framed and the complexity of the data display can determine whether the information gets used in decision-making, particularly for decisions that are difficult and unfamiliar, yet of importance to the individual (Hibbard et al., 2002; Vaiana and McGlynn, 2002). Furthermore, individuals may not be aware that the weight they place on a particular attribute, such as cost or quality, may not be accurately reflected in how they make their decisions (Hibbard et al., 2002). Edwards and Elwyn (2001) noted that stand-alone risk estimates can lead to overweighting low probabilities and underweighting high probabilities; framing the same risk information in terms of survival rather than mortality can affect perception and choice behaviors so that individuals have a more favorable impression of survival estimates (Tversky and Kahneman, 1981). In general, those attributes that are easy to assess, familiar, and have a precise frame of reference tend to get greater weight during decision-making than attributes that are less familiar or have a more fluid frame of reference. For example, in health plan decisions, costs may become a more important driver of choice because they are more familiar and precise than quality information, which is more complex and difficult for people to understand (Hibbard et al., 1997). In addition, integrating information on multiple attributes, such as costs and quality or side effects and quality-of-life, is challenging for individuals to tackle on their own, especially if tradeoffs are necessary to arrive at a final decision. Cognitive testing studies suggest that different ways of presenting the same information can be influential in changing how attributes or outcomes information are used in decision-making (Hibbard et al., 2002). Therefore, further research on efforts to help individuals gain greater familiarity in evaluating outcomes information and to identify information displays that facilitate this process will likely be very helpful for patient decision-making (Vaiana and McGlynn, 2002; Hibbard et al., 2002).

Physician Perspectives on Tailored Information for Patients

Physicians will likely welcome new technology that can help them tailor treatment recommendations to their patients' needs. Deber and Thompson (1987) noted that the main difference between physicians who recommended conservative breast surgery and those who recommended modified radical mastectomy for a hypothetical patient appeared to be their views on the relevancy of group-level results for individual patients. In their survey of 228 oncologists and surgeons, the authors found that physicians recommending aggressive treatments were more likely to agree with the statement: "Clinical trials do not allow the physician to take sufficient account of the uniqueness of the individual patient." Similarly, in a focus group study by Edwards et al. (1999), the physicians indicated that group-level information is less useful in clinical practice.

The importance of tailoring extends beyond the clinical characteristics of the patient. Physician participants in the Edwards et al. (1999) study also highlighted the need for a diversity of data presentation formats to tailor to the experience and comfort level of the patient. Physicians tended to view graphs as a good way to concretely present data (including both absolute and relative risks) without being too "scientific" or too time-consuming. However, they also recognized that graphic presentation might not work for all patients, some of whom may find chances or odds ratios more useful.

Data Banks or Data Bases

Opportunities and Challenges

The concept of using data banks or data bases to assist physicians in tailoring treatment recommendations for individual patients is not new. In his 1976 editorial, Fries suggested that data from patients closely matching the characteristics of the patient being seen by a physician be located in a data base. He gave an example listing characteristics of four patients with comparable clinical variables. For each patient, the 30 most similar patients were selected from the data base. Frequencies of adverse outcomes (e.g., mortality, rash) were presented along with the therapy associated with the best outcome. He noted that despite similar clinical characteristics, the data base produced four different prognoses and four different therapeutic recommendations. Hlatky et al. (1984) noted the complementary roles of data bases and randomized clinical trials, citing the importance of data bases for the vast majority of patients which randomized trials, with their stringent inclusion criteria, may not adequately represent.

However, concerns with the use of data bases have also been raised. Mantel (1983) cited the simple case in which the selectivity of treatment is often associated with disease severity, so that the most effective treatments may be given to the sickest patients—who in turn are most likely to suffer the worse outcomes, making the treatment appear to perform poorly. The idea of matching patient characteristics, as suggested by Fries (1976), may alleviate some of this problem. However, the size and balance of the pool of matching candidates and the consequent level of matching achieved in the data base would likely vary for patients with different characteristics and affect the reliability of the statistics produced. In fact, the reliability of the data base estimates would likely be lowest in extreme cases for whom available matching candidates is limited. For the data base to be useful as a decision aid, mechanisms for limiting selection and other forms of bias must be devised to ensure the reliability and representativeness of the information produced.

Data Bases as Decision Support

Published studies of the utility of data banks for decision support are rare. One study (Li et al., 1984) examined the influence of estimates from the Duke-Harvard Collaborative Coronary Artery Disease Data Bank on physicians' treatment recommendations. The authors found that physicians agreed on the recommended treatment course for 68 percent of the 60 patients and their recommendation for these patients rarely changed when presented with the estimates from the data bank. However, in the 19 patients for whom physicians' initial recommendations were divided, 10 percent of the recommendations did change. It is interesting to note that physicians who changed their recommendation subsequently placed greater value on the data bank, suggesting that physicians' perception of a decision or information aid may be improved if they feel that it can provide relevant new information for a clinical problem they faced.

Lessons from the Literature

The relevance of shared decision-making for clinical medicine has gained greater recognition in recent years. However, evidence suggests that patients are often not fully informed about treatment choices during the clinical encounter. Furthermore, the level of patient involvement in treatment decision-making is low. Contextual factors, such as the length of the patient-physician relationship, may influence the extent to which patients are involved. However, there is limited empirical evidence available to support this claim.

While patients' interest in treatment decision-making varies, their information needs are consistently high and they are likely to be active information seekers. Shared decision-making programs and decision aids offer opportunities to fulfill some of patients' need for information and decisional assistance. While continued evaluation of such aids is necessary, evidence to date suggests that they can increase patient knowledge, influence treatment decisions, and encourage patient involvement in decision-making, although their long-term effects are still unclear.

Research suggests that personalized information would most likely be popular among patients and physicians. Furthermore, individualized risk estimates are likely to be effective in influencing treatment choice. An outcomes data base offers a flexible strategy for providing individualized information to assist patients in treatment selection. However, several design issues should be considered:

- *Level of Patient and Physician Participation and Potential for Bias.* The level and selectivity of participation will directly affect the ability of the data base to provide unbiased individualized estimates. Therefore, it is important that the data base be inclusive of patients with different sociodemographic and clinical characteristics and of all available treatments, including watchful waiting.

- *Sample Size and Reliability of Estimates.* It will be important to assess how the number of matching candidates affects the quality of the information produced. Particularly if an individual's clinical characteristics are uncommon, the number of available matches may become quite low and the reliability of the estimates will deteriorate. It may be helpful to determine a threshold for matches below which estimates should not be considered useful.

- *Privacy and Confidentiality Concerns.* To enhance the breadth of participation and the cooperation of participants, it will be important to put in place safeguards to protect the confidentiality of patients and physicians who provide data for the data base.

- *Information Tailored to the Patient.* Patients prefer to see information that is personalized to their situation rather than generic results that may or may not apply to their unique profile. However, integrating information for multiple dimensions such as different side effects and quality-of-life outcomes is a difficult task. Therefore, it may be necessary to provide training or assistance to help patients and physicians develop skills and gain familiarity in incorporating different types of information during treatment decision-making.

- *Format and Content Considerations.* The ability of patients and clinicians to understand and use risk information can vary. Furthermore, their comfort level with different presentation formats (e.g., qualitative descriptions of risk, numeric estimates, graphical displays), also appears to vary. Therefore, it will be important to develop a flexible system of data presentation in which users can specify a mode of presentation and reading level with which they are comfortable. Creating options that allow a patient easy access to the information (e.g., at home via the computer or Internet) is likely to promote use; however, depending on the complexity of information shown, this may need to be balanced with information that is jointly reviewed and discussed by the patient and physician.

- *Cognitive Testing of Different Presentation Formats*. Research has shown that the weight given to different factors during decision-making can be influenced by presentation formats. It may be necessary to incorporate a cognitive testing stage to identify important presentation features that will facilitate the process of integrating information from multiple outcomes during decision-making.

- *Promotion of Data Base*. Use of the shared decision-making programs are influenced by patient and physician awareness of their availability. For the data base to achieve widespread use by the patient and clinical community, it will be important to actively promote or advertise the availability of the information, and this promotion will likely need to be ongoing.

- *Physician Attitudes and the Structure of the Patient Encounter Represent Potential Barriers that Must Be Addressed*. The current degree of information-sharing in clinical practice is poor, and physician attitudes of "knowing what is best for the patient" or "the information is too complex for the patient to fully grasp" are factors in the limited sharing of information that occurs today. Additionally, patient encounters are brief, hindering the ability of clinicians to take the time to fully educate their patients. These factors will need to be addressed if an informational data base is to achieve widespread use in clinical practice.

CHAPTER 4:
PROSTATE CANCER DATA BASE FEASIBILITY ASSESSMENT

Background

Prostate cancer is the most common form of non-skin cancer in men in the United States (American Cancer Society website, 2002) and is the second leading cause of cancer-related death among men in the United States (Jemal et al., 2002). The American Cancer Society (ACS) projects that in 2002, 189,000 new cases of prostate cancer will be diagnosed. Approximately 70 percent of all cases are diagnosed in men age 65 years and older. Prostate cancer is about twice as common in African-American men as in white men. The incidence of prostate cancer in the United States has increased over the last decade, owing to a combination of increased awareness among men and the use of serum PSA testing for early detection of prostate cancer.

As noted by the Prostate Cancer Outcomes Study (PCOS) group of the National Cancer Institute, patients with prostate cancer face uncertainty from many issues surrounding the management of the disease.

> It is not known, for instance, if the potential benefits of prostate cancer screening outweigh the risks, if surgery is better than radiation, or if treatment is better than no treatment in some cases. Decisions about treatments are also difficult to make … there are no randomized trials that compare the relative benefits of treating early-stage patients with radiation therapy, radical prostatectomy (surgical removal of the entire prostate gland along with nearby tissues), or watchful waiting. About 80 percent of men diagnosed with prostate cancer have early-stage disease. (National Cancer Institute PCOS website, 2002)

The therapeutic options for prostate cancer include watchful waiting, radical prostatectomy (surgery to remove the prostate), brachytherapy (radioactive seed implantation), external beam radiation, orchiectomy (removal of the testes) and androgen deprivation. Specific treatment—radiation therapy, radical prostatectomy, and hormonal therapies—can have serious effects on urinary, bowel, and sexual functions. Alternative treatments, such as diet modification, exist as well, although few alternative therapies have been evaluated. However, many patients with prostate cancer report using alternative treatments in concert with a traditional form of treatment.

Given the lack of clear scientific information to guide treatment choices for patients with prostate cancer, this condition was viewed by the study team and AHRQ as an excellent choice for assessing whether a national longitudinal prostate cancer outcomes data base would be a valuable tool to assist with treatment decisions and for evaluating the feasibility of creating such a data base.

The feasibility assessment consisted of identifying a set of questions to which patients and providers want answers (Appendix A), examining existing data bases and longitudinal data collection efforts in the area of prostate cancer, engaging providers and patients in a discussion of the utility of the data base concept and issues related to the feasibility of collecting and organizing data that could be used by patients and their physicians, and identifying key issues that should be considered in the design of a data base.

Consultative Meeting with Prostate Cancer Patient and Provider Representatives

We began the feasibility assessment with a set of one-on-one phone conversations with patients and/or representatives of patient groups and providers to explore the need for a People Like Me data base for prostate cancer, to explore what information was desired and where information gaps exist, and to identify existing data collection efforts that are tracking prostate cancer patients longitudinally. From these discussions, we identified a set of physicians and prostate cancer patient representatives whom we then invited to a one-day consultation meeting in Rockville, MD.

On March 22, 2002, RAND and AHRQ convened a group of 13 representatives (see Appendix C for a list of participants)—prostate cancer patients, prostate cancer advocates, and researchers and physicians who had been directly involved in collecting and disseminating information on outcomes of care. The purpose of the meeting was to obtain the input of potential end users—patients and providers—on the idea of developing a People Like Me outcomes data base on prostate cancer treatments and to explore major data base design issues. During the meeting, we asked the group to do the following:

- Define the important questions to which patients and providers want answers, so as to understand what data elements need to be captured and how many patients should be recruited to participate in the data base (see Appendix A).
- Define how the data would be used—what pieces of information are needed by whom and in what form.
- Evaluate how willing patients and/or providers would be to allow their data to be entered into the data base, under what conditions, and how potential barriers to participation might be addressed.

- Assess whether existing data bases provide a potential platform on which to build a national outcomes data base (could they be modified or enhanced?) and opportunities for collaboration (lessons learned).

- Discuss problems and challenges (e.g., confidentiality concerns, bias if full population of patients is not represented).

- Explore what entity would be a respected and trusted sponsor of such a data base.

For a portion of the meeting, participants were divided into two groups (patient/advocates and providers), and a RAND researcher led the discussion in each group. We decided to separate the patient and provider groups because we wanted each stakeholder group to have an opportunity to freely discuss the topics from its individual perspective. Below we summarize the discussion from this meeting.

Is There a Need for a National Outcomes Data Base for Prostate Cancer?

Overall, both the patient and provider representatives felt that a national prostate cancer outcomes data base would be of significant benefit to both patients and providers. The patient representatives indicated that it would be very helpful to be able to access information on various treatment options and side effects that fit their specific characteristics (e.g., age, race/ethnicity, stage of cancer). The patient group reinforced their belief that current access to information on prostate cancer and treatments is piecemeal at best and the information that is available is sometimes contradictory. The patient group also observed that the type of provider seen usually dictates the type of treatment recommended (i.e., urologists generally feel that radical prostetectomy is the best treatment course, whereas radiation oncologists lean toward radiation). Although many men diagnosed with prostate cancer know there are different treatments available, they are not sure where to turn to learn about the difference in outcomes for the various treatments. Uniformly, the patient advocates stated that a national data base would provide an independent place that patients and their families could turn to for up-to-date information that would help them make an informed decision on which type of treatment to pursue.

Providers generally felt that the data base would provide them with a tool to fill in knowledge gaps related to prostate cancer treatment, such as how certain people respond to treatments and/or how the treatment affects functional status and resumption of normal activities. In addition, a national data base might allow for unique populations to be identified, such as those with genetic predisposition to prostate cancer. Both groups agreed that a national outcomes data base would provide an important tool for shared decision-making between patients and providers, something that is currently lacking.

Existing Prostate Cancer Data Base Efforts—Do They Serve as a Starting Point?

A number of prostate cancer outcomes data bases have been created and are currently operational. During the meeting, representatives from three of these data base efforts—the Cancer of the Prostate Strategic Urologic Research Endeavor (CaPSURE), the Tri-Service military Center for Prostate Disease Research (CPDR) registry, and a hospital-based system at Memorial Sloan Kettering—gave brief descriptions of the content and uses of their data bases. CaPSURE collects data on prostate cancer treatment outcomes at 32 sites across the country and has over 8,000 men enrolled. CPDR (based at Walter Reed Medical Center) is a data base of over 16,000 men in 11 military hospitals. The third is a small and growing data base established by clinicians and researchers at Memorial Sloan Kettering and was designed to produce statistical prediction models to help guide treatment decisions. Detailed summaries of these data bases and other data collection efforts follow later in this chapter.

Although these data bases and others, such as the Surveillance, Epidemiology and End Results (SEER) program and the PCOS, are important tools for prostate cancer research, each is primarily geared to surveillance or research, and not to direct access by a patient's physician who is making decisions on their behalf. Currently, none of these data base efforts allow patients to directly access information or to tailor information from the data base to their specific characteristics to help guide decisions about treatment. So while much good information has been collected, little of it is being shared directly with patients who face the challenge of making treatment choices.

The discussion among the meeting participants also noted that each of the data bases has its own set of limitations, which prevents any single data base from serving as a platform or preexisting source of data to fully populate a People Like Me data base. All data bases would have to be modified. Examples of the limitations of existing data bases include

- missing subgroups of men (i.e., the poor, those with no health care, African-Americans, Asians, and those obtaining care from community practicing urologists)
- focusing on the initial course of treatment with no follow up information on subsequent courses of treatment or outcomes of care other than mortality (i.e., SEER)

- not capturing the full range of treatments by focusing data collection on urologists and not directly engaging radiation oncologists in the data collection
- focusing data collection on large centers of care and potentially missing a portion of the population that is different—both in patient characteristics and the type of treatment received in smaller communities
- not making data on outcomes directly available to patients or physicians for use in treatment decisions.

The Prostate Cancer Outcomes Study comes closest to capturing information on a representative sample of the population of prostate cancer patients; however, the data from this study could be better used to draw out important outcome information that could be shared with clinicians and patients.

Participants at the meeting agreed that the national outcomes data base could be modeled after these current data bases but should be expanded and would need to be made more patient friendly—specifically, that information from the data base would be made available to consumers and packaged for their use. Participants also noted that more information on pre- and posttreatment functional status is needed across all of the data collection efforts to determine the net effect of treatment, and that it would help if these assessments were standardized across the data bases to permit comparisons. Because there are variations across the different data collection efforts in the data elements collected, data definitions, and outcomes assessed, pooling of data from existing data collection efforts for the purposes of meta-analyses is also problematic.

What Information Is Needed?

During the meeting, we asked the two groups to comment on a draft set of questions an outcomes data base should focus on (see Appendix A). Overall, the physician and patient representatives agreed that the list of questions was appropriate. In particular, patient representatives expressed a desire for information on each step of the diagnosis and treatment process—for instance, what a rising PSA means, what the chances are of returning to pretreatment functioning, how the various treatments affect quality-of-life, and what treatments are available for complications/side effects of the cancer treatment.

Both groups agreed that a national prostate cancer data base would benefit patients and providers in terms of selecting treatment options and managing side effects. Both groups felt that although there is a great deal of information available on prostate cancer, many patients and providers do not have access to the most current information on the outcomes of various treatment options. For example, information on side effects and posttreatment functioning are based on follow-up studies from patients who were treated ten years ago, and these results may reflect very different practice styles and treatments than are currently used. Consequently, the quality-of-life outcomes of patients who were treated 10 years ago when there were fewer options available or when treatments were more invasive, are not necessarily applicable to patients undergoing treatment today.

Both groups agreed that data are not available on how prostate cancer treatment affects general aspects of functioning and quality-of-life, such as being able to complete normal daily living activities and returning to work (Volk et al., 1999). Most data currently available focus on urinary/bowel dysfunction and sexual dysfunction. Patients who had undergone treatment stated that they did not realize that it could take up to a year to recover to pretreatment functioning and they were under the impression that it would take a matter of weeks. In addition, in terms of treatment success, patients want information on gauging how successful their treatment is in terms of functioning (i.e., what constitutes successful treatment). For example, if a patient is suffering from postsurgery incontinence, how many pads per day is normal for a patient who has been "successfully" treated? Finally, patients stated a desire to be able to learn who the top physicians are who perform prostate cancer procedures. Patients expressed a desire to make an educated decision on whom to see for the various treatment procedures (surgery, hormonal therapy, radiation). They wanted to know which doctors and which hospitals had done the largest volume of procedures, and—optimally—what the outcomes of care were for patients treated by different physicians.

Participation, Sponsorship, and Data Collection

There was consensus between both groups that a prostate cancer data base would be useful for both patients and providers and that data should be collected with input from both patients and providers. The patient group did not feel it would be difficult to get men to agree to participate and that confidentiality would not be an issue. One patient advocate had done an informal survey of over 100 men from a local prostate cancer support group: All agreed that a national data base is needed and would be beneficial, and that they would participate without hesitation. When asked who should sponsor such a data base, the patient group agreed that it should be a nonpolitical, highly visible, trusted body, such as the American Cancer Society.

When asked how the information in a national data base should be collected and accessed, many agreed that a Web-based design would be good, but that it might miss groups of men, such as those who are not computer literate and those who do not have access to a computer. Patients thought that a multifaceted approach to gathering and

42

providing information, such as through the computer and through written materials, would be best.

The most important aspect of a national prostate cancer data base, as cited by both patients and providers, is that it would provide a tool by which both patients and providers could make an informed, shared decision on which treatment options are best for a particular patient. This decision would be based on the patient's age, state of cancer, PSA, Gleason score,[1] grade of biopsy, and comorbidities. Patients would be able to evaluate differences in functional outcomes of various treatments by patient race, income, and geographic area.

Summary of Existing Outcomes Data Bases

CaPSURE.net

Overview

The Cancer of the Prostate Strategic Urologic Research Endeavor (CaPSURE) is a research project managed by the Urology Outcomes Research Group of the University of California at San Francisco (UCSF) Department of Urology. It is sponsored financially by TAP Pharmaceuticals. The project has built a data base that collects longitudinal data on prostate cancer patients located across the United States. The data base collects information on treatment outcomes and the impact of prostate cancer on a patient's quality-of-life. Researchers and policy makers at UCSF use the data base to evaluate outcomes of prostate cancer. Information is fed back electronically to physician participants in the study to track how their patients and practice patterns compare to those of other urologists. In some cases, although this is not the norm, physicians report using the information with their patients to help make treatment decisions.

Patients were first enrolled in the data base in 1995, and all data collected between 1995 and 1999 were manually collected and entered. In 1999, data entry and access to the data base became Web-based. This allowed for more patients to participate without substantially increasing costs. It also gave physicians the ability to see their patients' data and compare it to national data in real time.

---

[1] A Gleason Score is a grading system used by pathologists to describe the appearance of the prostate cancer tissue. It provides the physician with information to make estimates regarding the length of survival following a diagnosis of prostate cancer, and is generally combined with a patient's PSA level and clinical stage to make a survival estimate. The Gleason grading system is based exclusively on the architectural pattern of the glands of the prostate tumor. It evaluates how effectively the cells of any particular cancer are able to structure themselves into glands resembling those of the normal prostate (a tumor whose structure is nearly normal—well differentiated—will probably have a biological behavior relatively close to normal). The grading system runs from grade 1 (very well differentiated) to grade 5 (very poorly differentiated). Grades 1 and 2 closely resemble normal prostate cancer cells whereas grade 5 usually predicts a poor prognosis. The Gleason Score is the result of summing two Gleason grades from different specimens. Thus the lowest possible Gleason Score is 2 and the highest possible is 10.

Currently, 8,100 patients are enrolled in the data base, and about 1,500 new patients enroll each year, a number that is constrained by the budget. Approximately 5 percent of the patients drop out each year. Physicians at 32 practice sites participate in the study by entering their patients' clinical data into the data base. Nurses and other clinic staff also assist in the task of entering clinical data. The majority of physicians participating in the project are urologists, so the data base is heavily weighted toward patients who undergo surgery. The practice sites are located throughout the country; however, the patients and physicians within the CaPSURE sites do not represent the population of patients receiving care for prostate cancer or the population of physicians and facilities that provide care to prostate cancer patients. The vast majority of data contained in the data base come from urologists in selected practice sites, and the inclusion of radiation oncology information and patients who undergo this treatment is limited.

Data Base Components

The data base contains two types of information: (1) clinical data on patients and (2) patient-reported data on quality-of-life. Physicians and staff at the participating clinics enter clinical data for individual patients onto a password-protected secure web-server hosted by a third party (NetOutcomes). The clinical data collected include demographic information, method of cancer diagnosis, clinical pathological staging, PSA values, Gleason scores, treatment choices, and various lab results. The website for the data base has several features that enable the physician to do analyses on the patients' data and compare it to national data. The analyses are displayed in graphical formats and do permit subgroup analyses (such as demographics, and diagnosis and staging).

CaPSURE also contains patient-reported data on quality-of-life issues from semiannual mailed surveys. The quality-of-life issues that are addressed in the surveys include treatment side effects, such as urinary, bowel, and sexual function, satisfaction with treatment, fear of recurrence, physical functioning, bodily pain, general health, fatigue, social functioning, and mental health. Researchers and site management staff at UCSF manage the quality-of-life survey process. The data from returned surveys is de-identified before it is transmitted to the third-party web host and made available to physicians. Therefore, physicians see only aggregate quality-of-life data provided by all patients in the clinic, rather than an individual patient's responses. As with the clinical data, the data base offers several analysis functions so that physicians can compare quality-of-life information for all patients in their clinic with national data.

By viewing the information within the data base, physicians can show patients information about side effects associated with the different types of treatment. They can also look at the characteristics of patients who receive a particular type of treatment, but because the data base does not include radiation oncologists as a primary source of data, their patients are underrepresented in the data base. The semiannual survey asks patients to report on whether they used some type of complementary or alternative medicine to treat their cancer, though it does not capture detailed information to examine what alternative therapies are being used and with what effect. About 30 percent of the patients in the data base report that they use some type of complementary or alternative medicine.

Physician Participation

The physician sites that participate in CaPSURE are a convenience sample of urology practices. In the first two years of the project, the study team recruited sites known to have large urology practices and also included sites from the members of the project's advisory group (whose urologists were interested in the study). Once the program became operational and known, the recruitment effort largely shifted to a strategy where urology practice sites self-identified themselves as being interested in joining the project. The CaPSURE team then selected the sites on the basis of their ability to recruit patients and their geographic or site diversity. There has been growing interest among urologists in participation in the CaPSURE data base. In the past three years, the major selection criteria have focused on filling gaps in site, ethnic, and geographic variation to increase participants from the Rocky Mountain and Midwest regions.

When a clinic is selected to participate in CaPSURE, all physicians who treat prostate cancer patients at the clinic are invited to participate in the data base project, though not all of them do. Physicians are paid $150.00 for each new patient they recruit, and they receive $100 annually for each continuing patient. This payment does not fully cover the costs to the physician for participating, indicating that the participating physicians have a strong interest in the goals of the project.

Physicians use the information in the CaPSURE data base in a variety of ways. They can obtain aggregated summaries on patients in their clinic or aggregated summaries on all current and former participating sites. According to the UCSF staff, physician have used the information in their discussions with patients, although on a limited basis.

Patient Characteristics and Recruitment

Physicians and clinic staff at each practice site recruit patients who fit certain eligibility criteria. To be eligible to participate, patients must have a new, biopsy-confirmed prostate cancer diagnosis. Participating patients must provide written consent before being enrolled in the data base. If patients decline to participate, only limited demographic information is entered into the data base for research purposes (to compare participants to nonparticipants). Patients have the choice of participating in the project at different levels. They can consent to having only their clinical data collected, or they can choose to only complete the quality-of-life surveys, or they can consent to both. After treatment is completed, patients still receive the quality-of-life surveys every six months, regardless of whether or not they are still receiving medical care from the participating clinic. The average length of enrollment has been 36 months, although the length of time continues to increase.

There is a strong effort to include a diverse set of patients in the data base, though this has been a continuing challenge to researchers. Currently, 10 - 12 percent of the patients in the data base are African-American. The data base contains few Latino and Asian men. The patient survey is available in English and Spanish; no other patient group in the data base is large enough to justify the cost or effort to translate the survey into any other language. The average age of patients in the data base is 60 years old. Patients receive no payment for participating, but they do benefit by receiving information about prostate cancer research through a newsletter and by accessing publications online.

Online Format

The data base is accessible through a website that was developed by NetOutcomes. NetOutcomes is responsible for maintaining the website and data base and responding to all technical assistance inquiries from participating sites. Researchers at UCSF receive customized data sets from NetOutcomes on a quarterly basis.

The CaPSURE.net website has four major functions: (1) data entry; (2) clinic graphs; (3) research; and (4) site management. In the data entry area, individual patients can be found by specifying any of the following: doctor's name, the patient's first or last name, patient ID, patient medical record, patient date of birth. New patients can also be added. Once a patient is found, summaries of the following can be displayed: status, clinic visit, labs and imaging, prostate biopsy pathology, surgery and treatments, medications, erectile dysfunction, clinical trial, survey pathology, hospitalization summary.

The "clinic graphs" area of the website displays aggregate outcomes and demographics under the following headings: demographics, diagnosis and staging, treatment, recurrence and survival, and quality-of-life. These subareas are called "grouped patients analyses." Most display outcomes and demographics as bar charts. The exception is "Quality-of-Life," where percentages are plotted over time. Time is measured as months since treatment. For all grouped patient analyses, it is possible to graph either data for the individual clinic, for the aggregate data set, or for both. It is also possible to show a subset of the clinic data to display only outcome for one doctor. Most of the reports are "fixed" in their basic design but allow the end-user some flexibility to specify and create comparisons of interest.

Each grouped patient analysis consists of individual patient analyses. Treatment analyses include these individual analyses: initial treatment, prostatectomy method, hormonal therapy, luteinizing hormone–releasing hormone (LHRH) agonist use, anti-androgen use, and irradiation method. Quality-of-life consists of these individual analyses: urinary function, bowel function, sexual function, satisfaction with treatment, satisfaction with care, fear of recurrence, physical function, bodily pain, general health, vitality, fatigue, social function, and mental health.

Further subsetting of the clinic data is possible depending on the individual patient analysis chosen. For example, if one chooses "Protastectomy Method" under the treatment analysis group, the data can be analyzed by insurance status, age at diagnosis, PSA at diagnosis, Gleason score, or tumor node metastatis stage. It is possible to display outcomes by conditioning on individual categories for any combination of these variables.

Operational Aspects and Costs

Currently, TAP Pharmaceuticals provides all funding for CaPSURE and owns the data contained in the data base. It does not own the data base software or data base development. The data base management is outsourced to NetOutcomes. NetOutcomes developed the CaPSURE.net interface and worked with the project's researchers to convert the data base to the online format. Researchers at UCSF receive data dumps from NetOutcomes once every three months for the purposes of conducting research. TAP Pharmaceuticals is not involved in the research efforts.

Cleaning and pre-processing the data address problems arising from changes to specifications over time (common to longitudinal studies), shortcomings in the data base design (e.g. duplicate observations, missed opportunities for input validation), and different variable names used by UCSF programmers from those used in the data base.

Because they do not own the data base design, researchers at UCSF and TAP Pharmaceuticals have limited influence on design changes.

Costs to the project include labor for the UCSF staff, payments to NetOutcomes for hosting the data base and website on its server, and payments to the participating sites and physicians. We were unable to get an estimate of NetOutcome's costs for its role in the project. A low estimate of the annual costs to UCSF is $3.5 million. The project budget provided by TAP Pharmaceuticals strictly determines how many patients can be enrolled in the data base. Since the sites enroll new patients each year, the costs for the sites are always increasing. Determining how many patients to enroll based on the budget can be difficult because the dropout rate throughout the year is unknown. UCSF is currently holding the enrollment of new patients to 1,500 per year.

Staffing

Coordinating and maintaining the CaPSURE data base require a multidisciplinary staff at several organizations. Staffing for the project includes employees of TAP Pharmaceuticals (the sponsor), the UCSF Urology Outcomes Research Group, and NetOutcomes.

The CaPSURE staff at UCSF comprises two teams, with 8-10 people on each team. One team includes the researchers who set research priorities for the project and determine what needs to be included in the CaPSURE data base. This team includes several SAS programmers, statistical consultants, three urologists who provide clinical expertise about prostate cancer, and researchers who conduct a variety of studies. One of the SAS programmers is an experienced data base programmer who supports the data transition from the data base at NetOutcomes to the needs of several SAS programmers at UCSF. His expertise is critical, in particular given that the NetOutcomes software is proprietary. Without this programmer at UCSF, data quality would suffer greatly, although this might not become obvious to the public, because data quality is not easy to measure.

The other UCSF team is a site management team and comprises 8 – 10 staff members. This team is involved in all aspects of managing the participating sites and spends a large part of their time on work related to the semiannual mailed patient surveys. Approximately four months out of the year is spent working on the surveys. The team is responsible for everything involved in the production and mailing of the survey, with the exception of printing, which is outsourced. The team also manages the survey data collection process. They track the returned surveys and follow up with patients if there are any questionable responses, including problems with illegible handwriting. When a survey is returned, the team scans the surveys into a computer to create an electronic form of the survey, de-identifies it, and transmits the data to NetOutcomes. NetOutcomes then enters the survey data into the data base and makes them available to physicians.

Converting to Web-based data collection for the patient survey would significantly reduce project costs and eliminate problems caused by illegible handwriting. However, the patient population at this time lacks sufficient access to the Internet and/or interest in completing the survey online. As access to the Internet increases and the patient population becomes more comfortable using the Web, providing the survey online will be revisited. Another factor that will need to be considered in evaluating the merits of shifting to online administration of the survey is the access speed of the Internet connections of patients being asked to complete the survey; patients with slower phone modem access may be unwilling to complete the survey online depending on its design.

NetOutcomes also has several staff members devoted to working on the CaPSURE data base, although the exact number is unclear. These employees also have a diverse set of skills, including data base management, website design, and usability testing. NetOutcomes is also responsible for responding to all technical assistance questions from the participating sites.

Challenges and Future Directions

The CaPSURE project, along with most prostate cancer outcomes data bases, faces several challenges to being able to give highly personalized information about the range of prostate cancer treatments and outcomes to all patients. First, the data base is not representative of all the providers of treatment; in particular, radiation oncologists are a minority in the data base because the clinical sites targeted are urology practices. CaPSURE also does not have much penetration in the Rocky Mountain states, and represents a narrow swath of clinic sites. Additionally, the patient population is fairly homogeneous, both in terms of treatments and limited enrollment by minority populations. Each of these factors reduces the generalizability of the information. Staff at UCSF seem interested in making the data base accessible to patients in the future but note that much work is required to determine what information should be provided and the format for doing so.

SEER Data Base

Overview

The Surveillance, Epidemiology and End Results (SEER) Program of the National Cancer Institute collects a wide range of information on all types of cancers diagnosed in the United States. Prostate cancer is one of the many cancers included in the SEER data base. The data in the SEER data base come from population-based cancer registries that represent approximately 26 percent of patients with cancer in the United States. Though national in scope, the data base is not truly representative of all cancer patients in the United States.

The registry seeks to collect information on all cancer diagnoses that occur among residents within a geographical area. The data comes from a variety of sources including hospitals, physicians, and laboratories. Any health care provider or facility that serves patients who live in a registry area is mandated to provide data on residents' cancer diagnoses. The majority of data comes from hospitals and is collected from claims data and medical record reviews. Because the SEER data base population is based on the residents in the SEER registry area, data may also be collected from hospitals and providers in neighboring states.

The number of registries has fluctuated since the SEER program began in 1973. Registries currently operate in Kentucky, Greater California, Louisiana, New Jersey, Georgia (rural areas plus Atlanta), Connecticut, Iowa, New Mexico, Utah, Hawaii, American Indians in Arizona, Alaskan natives in Alaska, and the Seattle-Puget Sound area. Recently, SEER has expanded its data collection to cover additional regions in an effort to address gaps in populations reflected in the data base.

The SEER registry tracks individual cancer diagnoses rather than individual patients. In other words, a patient is added to the registry when he or she gets an initial primary diagnosis of cancer in one area of the body. If the same person receives a primary diagnosis of cancer in another area of the body at a later time, the patient enters the data base again as a second case. Therefore, the registry may contain more than one cancer case for a single individual. It is not known how many actual people the registry represents.

The SEER registry conducts annual follow up for vital status only. Because the registry provides survival statistics, follow up with patients is continued until their death. The SEER program primarily gets data on date and cause of death from state death certificates. It also sometimes retrieves this information from Medicare sources through the Social Security administration. The validity of data from state death certificates and cause of death determination has been discussed and questioned in the scientific literature.

The SEER data base makes data on cancer incidence, mortality, and survival rates available in a public-use data file. There currently are data on three million in situ and invasive cancer cases, and approximately 170,000 cases are added to the registry each year. The data available to the public are usually two years old and are de-identified to protect the identity of patients.

The annual budget for SEER is $25 million, which covers the registry staff as well as roughly 15 staff (not all working on SEER full-time) within the National Cancer Institute's Statistics Branch who conduct statistical analyses of the data.

Data Base Components, Uses, and Limitations

The data base contains demographic data (age, gender, race), primary tumor site, morphology, age at diagnosis, stage of cancer at time of diagnosis, first course of treatment, and survival rates within each stage of cancer. It does not contain information on the details of treatment and whether subsequent treatment is provided to a patient, pretreatment clinical characteristics of the patient, and patient functioning before and after treatment. The sole outcome variable in SEER is survival.

The SEER data base is a valuable source of data for such clinical information as incidence and survival rates. SEER can also provide information on characteristics of people who choose a certain type of treatment. However, it cannot provide more qualitative information about side effects and impact on quality-of-life based on a patient's treatment choice. To accomplish this, the National Cancer Institute and other organizations use SEER data to perform additional research. Some of these studies are called SEER Rapid Response Special Studies. One of the largest of these studies is the Prostate Cancer Outcomes Study, sponsored by the National Cancer Institute.

Another major project using the SEER data base has linked the data in the registry to Medicare claims data. The SEER-Medicare data provide valuable longitudinal information about cancer diagnosis, treatment, and follow up. They can be an especially good source of information on acute and chronic complications of cancer treatments. The data have been linked multiple times, first in 1991, and then in 1995 and 1999. Data linkage with Medicare data was accomplished for 93 percent of people in the SEER data base who are 65 years or older. The SEER-Medicare data linkage is a valuable resource for prostate cancer information. The generalizability of all the data in the SEER-Medicare data base is being studied and should be considered when reporting the data, particularly for cancers that have lower incidence in older age groups. Although extensive efforts are taken to de-identify SEER-Medicare data, a potential for identification remains, and thus, the data are not available to the public.

Patient Characteristics and Recruitment

Patients in the registry area who receive a primary cancer diagnosis are automatically entered into the SEER data base. They are not given the option of opting out. The registries are dispersed throughout the country and some registries were

51

specifically established with the goal of increasing minority representation in the data base. SEER data on race is collected from medical records and registration information. Hispanic ancestry is collected as a separate variable and is identified by applying an algorithm to detect Spanish surnames. SEER's race data for patients who are not African-American or white are less valid, and none of the SEER race data have been externally validated.

Staffing

Each SEER registry employs 20 - 40 full-time employees, who are responsible for collecting the data for the registry. Staff at the National Cancer Institute, including administrators and researchers, also work for the SEER program.

Prostate Cancer Outcomes Study

Overview

The Prostate Cancer Outcomes Study provides important information on quality-of-life and treatment outcomes for prostate cancer patients. The National Cancer Institute (NCI) began conducting PCOS in 1994. The study collects data from patient surveys and medical records. Patients were recruited from SEER cancer registries in Connecticut, Utah, New Mexico, Atlanta, Los Angeles, and Seattle. Over 11,000 men were eligible for the study because they had been diagnosed with biopsy-confirmed primary invasive prostate cancer between October 1, 1994 and October 31, 1995. From this study population, 5,672 men were sampled and 3,533 completed the six-month survey, 12-month survey, or both. Eighty-three percent of the men who were eligible to complete the 24-month follow up survey did so. Ninety-nine percent of the 3,533 men had their medical records abstracted. The study sought to generate a representative sample in terms of age, race, geography, health care setting, and treatment choices. Certain age and racial/ethnic groups were over-sampled, though the entire study focused primarily on white non-Hispanic, Hispanic, and African-American men. This is a strength of this data base that was made possible by building off of the SEER data.

Quality-of-life surveys were sent to participating patients at six, 12, and 18 months after their diagnosis. The surveys were available in Spanish. Follow up is done annually to check on vital status and address changes, and to provide a patient newsletter. In fall 1999, a five-year follow up survey was conducted, and the potential exists to conduct a ten-year follow up survey as well. PCOS also includes data from patients' medical records, such as patients' PSA scores, clinical stage and grade, treatments, and specific hormone therapies given. Data on age at diagnosis, race/ethnicity, clinical stage and grade of tumor, and the initial treatment choice came from SEER. Education and income data were mapped from Census data, matching by zip code blocks.

The PCOS survey focuses on the impact of prostate cancer treatment on urinary, sexual, and bowel function. The treatment options that it focuses on are surgery, radiation therapy, and hormone therapy. The study data can tell a variety of things about what kinds of treatments patients with certain characteristics are choosing, as well as the side effects that are experienced by patients who choose those treatments. Although the PCOS survey asks patients whether or not they engage in alternative therapies (e.g., dietary changes, herbal supplements, exercise), NCI is not evaluating the relationship between these supplemental therapies and treatment outcomes or quality-of-life.

The results that have emerged from analyses of the PCOS longitudinal tracking data underscore the potential value of developing People Like Me outcomes data bases. Some of the completed research has found important differences in the side effects experienced by patients who choose different treatments. Another study has found that PSA levels, Gleason scores, and age are the best predictors of the spread of the disease outside the prostate. Analysis of the PCOS data also show that age at diagnosis, pretreatment health status, comorbidity, and treatment choice are the most important factors contributing to patient outcomes-covariates that a People Like Me data base would want to use to display differential outcomes tailored to the demographic and clinical characteristics of patients. Each of the analyses derived from PCOS data lends credence to the need to capture information on outcomes by different clinical and demographic characteristics of the patient. However, the information gleaned from the PCOS analyses is not being communicated directly to patients and doctors in a way that promotes shared decision-making at the point of care; so while PCOS realizes part of the vision of a People Like Me data base, it has not taken the additional step of creating an information tool for use by patients and physicians.

Staffing, Operational Aspects, and Costs

The staff for the PCOS study include four people at the National Cancer Institute and an unknown number of people who work with the six SEER registries involved in the study. The PCOS staff at NCI performed the study under contract, rather than as a grant, which provided some cost-savings. To recruit and track approximately 3,500 patients, PCOS has spent an estimated $7 - 10 million since 1994.

Challenges and Future Directions

One way to make better use of the PCOS data is to increase efforts to disseminate the results directly to patients—although work is required to understand how to do this effectively. Furthermore, PCOS has not focused much activity on dissemination and does not know how results of its studies have affected practice behavior.

A PCOS staff member noted that much could be done to repackage existing information and disseminate it more effectively to patients. This would involve determining which People Like Me questions have already been answered or could be answered by the existing data bases, grading this evidence, and determining where the information gaps are and how best to fill them.

It was also noted that it would be valuable to jointly agree on common definitions for the variables that are being collected across data bases. A factor hindering the pooling of data across these collection efforts is that elements are difficult to compare because of differing definitions used and outcomes tracked.

Center for Prostate Disease Research Tri-Service Multicenter Prostate Patient Data Base Registry

Overview

The Center for Prostate Disease Research (CPDR) Tri-Service Multicenter Registry collects information about prostate cancer from men in the TriCare military hospital system. The data base captures information from the major military hospital centers nationally. The data base collects clinical data, complications, and limited quality-of-life information from men with diagnosed cases of prostate cancer and those who have clinical indicators of prostate cancer risk (i.e., elevated PSA scores but no positive biopsy of cancer).

Unlike those data bases that have been developed in the nonmilitary sector, the nature of the military organization reinforces physician participation in the project and also contributes to the high level of participation and compliance by the patients. For men who meet the clinical criteria for inclusion, 99 percent agree to participate in the registry. Within the military system, active duty personnel must be seen by a physician twice a year. These biannual visits allow CPDR to capture ongoing information about patients who have prostate cancer or are at elevated risk. Retirees are not seen as often, but these individuals still maintain fairly regular contact with the military hospital system to receive care, which facilitates tracking patients longitudinally.

CPDR has adopted a participatory model in its design and operation. At each hospital site, CPDR enlists physicians to become collaborators on the research team, so that there is active commitment to and participation by all sites in the data base. Physicians within each of the participating hospital sites are encouraged to request data from the data base for their own research and to publish their findings. The TriCare system has successfully integrated the project into the clinical setting and even uses it to help maintain contact with patients and involve them in their care. The data are used to generate short monthly reports at the hospital site level to use in tracking and managing patients.

The data base officially started in 1994 and collected data from only one military hospital at that time. Up to as many as 13 military hospitals have participated since the project's inception. The current number of participating sites is 11 and includes 16,025 patients. The hospitals are all located in large cities; small military hospitals located in small cities or more rural settings are not participating in the data base. CPDR does not have information on the nonparticipating sites to assess whether there are key differences in the populations (e.g., age) at participating and nonparticipating hospitals. CPDR does receive requests from other hospital sites that are not participating to join the registry program; however, CPDR does not have funding to support expansion of the registry to other sites.

Until 1999, the only patients enrolled in the data base were men with diagnoses of prostate cancer. Beginning in 1999, the data base expanded to include patients with elevated PSA levels. CPDR is interested in tracking these patients who are considered at elevated risk because approximately 80 percent of them will have active prostate cancer at some later point in time. As of June 2002, approximately 16,025 patients were enrolled in the data base. Of these, approximately 12,000 have an active case of prostate cancer; the remaining 4,000 patients in the data base have an elevated PSA level with a benign biopsy.

Data Base Components

The CPDR data base is a relational Oracle data base. The data base is not directly accessible through the Web or by other means. At this time, there is no mechanism in place for physicians or anyone else to be able to get data in real time.

CPDR collects general and prostate cancer-specific data, such as age, race, PSA levels, tumor differentiation, Gleason scores, and staging information. The data base contains approximately 500 data fields in 48 tables that include registration, patient contact information, pretreatment diagnosis, cancer staging, treatment types, follow up and recurrence, quality-of-life issues, and many others. There are detailed data tables for each type of cancer treatment. Data are collected for standard clinical care, which includes hormonal therapy, radiation therapy, chemotherapy, and surgery. Each major treatment type has a subset of questions asked. The majority of the information in the data base is collected during the treatment stage.

Data for the prostate data base is obtained from three different sources. The primary source is the military's Composite Health Care System (CHCS) data base, an electronic data base that collects comprehensive medical information (laboratory and pathology values, pharmacy, treatments, etc.) about all patients within the TriCare System. It contains demographic information about each patient, as well as some specific clinical information about all health conditions. Rather than asking the providers to enter the same data twice, CPDR imports data relevant for the prostate data base directly from the CHCS. The CHCS captures nearly all the data CPDR requires; however, it is supplemented by additional data collection from two other sources.

The second source of data is clinical notes in the patients' charts. Each physician is required to maintain a hard-copy chart for a patient in addition to the CHCS electronic data record. Clinical data come only from the provider and not from the patient. The clinical data are collected by on-site data managers in each hospital who review the medical charts and manually enter information into the CPDR data base.

The third source of data is patient surveys that primarily focus on quality-of-life issues, although to date these have been limited in scope. CPDR views patient-reported data as subjective in nature and relies more on clinical assessment from the two previously discussed sources. Patients fill out a baseline survey at their first visit (either elevated PSA or actual positive biopsy of cancer, but pretreatment). The survey collects information on family history and clinical issues, such as PSA level, and pretreatment sexual, urinary, and bowel function, and other quality-of-life issues. Once treatment has commenced, patients are surveyed annually during their visits to the hospital. If a patient has not been seen for over a year, the data manager will mail the survey to him. The survey is a component of the project's efforts to keep patients engaged in the longitudinal data collection by prompting patients to make an appointment with the urologist. If a patient says that he would like to make an appointment, the data manager will contact the patient directly to make the appointment and get him into the system for reassessment.

Survey responses are entered into the data base, and the hard copy of the survey is attached to the medical record. Because patients are seen so frequently and this population is very compliant in making and showing up for appointments, the mailed survey is not seen as a major source of information for the data base. Rather, the focus is on gathering information for the data base during the clinical visit because data managers typically get more complete information from patients during their medical appointments. The mailed survey is 16 pages long and considered burdensome for patients to complete; it is undergoing revision to reduce its length and to capture a broader set of data on the patient's functional status. The project staff meets annually to discuss the project, including possible changes to the survey.

The data base does not routinely collect information on alternative treatments, although physicians are free to note this in an open data field. Data on the use of alternative therapies are not included in the reports to physicians and are not used for research. The primary reason for excluding the capture of information on alternative treatments from the registry is the difficulty of developing standardized definitions of alternative treatments, which makes it difficult to compare alternative treatment outcomes.

Patient Characteristics and Recruitment

All of the men in the data base have either an active case of prostate cancer or an elevated PSA level. Patients can only be recruited for the project if they receive care from one of the 11 participating military hospital facilities. Most of the patients in the data base are in the military or retired from the military, although civilians who receive care at participating facilities can also participate. All participants provide written consent.

The average age of patients at the time of enrollment is 61. The average length of enrollment is 5 - 6 years, and the reasons for dropping out of the data base are varied. Many men drop out when their cancer is in remission and they are no longer receiving any treatment. Surveys are still sent to data base participants regardless of their health status. Deceased patients are dropped from active participation in the data base. CPDR's goal is to maintain contact with the men in the data base indefinitely.

The data base does not collect information on the income level of participants, but because they receive military benefits, it is unlikely that a significant number of men in the data base are below poverty level. The data base is likely to be somewhat more representative of all income levels, because treatment for military servicemen is free, and thus cost is not a barrier to patients seeking and receiving care. As a result, the CPDR data base is likely to include more low-income patients, compared to private-sector data bases. Another advantage of the TriCare System is that men within the system can see any provider they would like. Approximately 17 - 18 percent of the patients in the data base are African-American. Because of the United States military presence in the Philippines, Filipino men are well represented in the data base, but other Asian groups are not. The data base contains few Hispanics. There are some Native Americans in the data base, but the numbers are too small for group-specific analyses.

Physician Participation

Because of the unique characteristics of the military setting, the cooperation of the physicians is expected and financial incentives to participate are prohibited. CPDR has taken steps to engage physicians in each of the hospital sites to be co-partners in the data collection and research activities of CPDR. In addition to establishing co-investigator roles for physicians in all sites, CPDR holds annual meetings with the clinicians to discuss data fields, to address problems/questions, and to assist with data analysis for research.

CPDR is actively committed to ensuring that the data base is relevant for physicians to use in improving the care that they deliver to patients with prostate cancer. Physicians use the data within the data base to help make treatment decisions and to compare their clinic's performance with other participating facilities within the TriCare system. Each month, CPDR sends providers a hard-copy report that summarizes site-level data. The report provides information on their own patients' progress, and physicians can use it to compare outcomes across different sites (but not across different physicians at their own site). This can help motivate physicians to provide better care. Physicians can submit a request to CPDR to get data for individual patients for use when making treatment decisions. The data can be put in a graphical format and used in discussions with the patient, although this does not occur with great frequency.

Physicians and/or staff automatically inform the on-site CPDR data managers about patient appointments with registry patients, and they give data managers access to the patient charts. Some providers participate actively in the project by using the data base to conduct their own research. However, most physicians never request additional data from the data base.

It should be noted, however, that CPDR currently is not set up to provide patients direct access to the information to compare treatment options and outcomes. While this has been discussed as a possible long-term goal, CPDR is concerned about a range of issues including legal problems in making patient data public (Institutional Review Board concerns about protecting patient privacy) and that statistics may be old and may not predict a patient's real problem. It is likely that if patients had access to the data at some point in the future, CPDR would be required to re-consent existing patients in the data base, which would be extremely burdensome and difficult to do. At this point, information from the system is provided to patients in a more neutral fashion, by sending patients reminders or prompts to have their PSA checked and, in some cases, by physicians as they counsel their patients.

Staffing

Several groups of staff members play a role in managing and using the data base. Physicians participate in the data base project by helping to identify patients who should be recruited into the project. The majority of participating physicians are urologists and medical oncologists.

Data managers are CPDR employees who work on-site at the participating facilities. They represent the data base project in the clinical setting and play a major role. There are currently 18 data managers working at the 11 facilities (1 - 3 managers per site). Most data managers have a medical background. They are responsible for recruiting patients, securing patients' written consent, providing health education support to patients and their families, performing data entry, transmitting data to the central data base on a daily basis, assisting principal investigators with data requests, and serving as the local representative for the project to the Institutional Review Board (IRB). The health education that they provide to patients about prostate cancer comes from the CPDR data base and the National Cancer Institute. While consulting with patients, the data managers present the prostate cancer information in a neutral way to avoid influencing patients to choose one type of treatment course over another.

The on-site data manager contacts all men who receive care from one of the participating military hospitals and who meet the study criteria. The data manager meets with each of these patients, describes the data base project, and encourages the patient to participate. Patients must provide written consent in order for their data to be collected for the data base.

There are many benefits to having the data managers work on-site. They can recruit patients at the start of their diagnosis and treatment to capture important baseline information for assessing outcomes. They can respond quickly to identify and recruit eligible patients, and because of the regularity of patient encounters with the military health system, they have frequent access to patients to perform follow up assessments.

The other project staff members are CPDR employees who maintain the data base and provide data to the hospital sites. CPDR also provides technical assistance to the sites and meets with data managers and principal investigators on an annual basis to discuss the project and make any necessary changes to the protocol or survey. CPDR employees play an important role in ensuring the quality of the data within the data base. CPDR staff identify missing data and data with errors using a manual technique as well as with a software package integrated into the data base. They notify the data managers, who are then responsible for doing necessary follow up and correcting errors.

Military medical residents assist in this process. Every effort is made to have complete, accurate data, though sometimes it is not entirely possible.

Operational Aspects and Costs

The CPDR receives approximately $2 million per year from the federal government through the Nery M. Jackson Foundation for the Advancement of Military Medicine to operate the data base. CPDR receives an additional three to four grants per year, which total between $500,000 and $1 million. The budget pays for the CPDR staff salaries and the salaries of the on-site data managers. The budget also covers the costs of providing data to the study's principal investigators, reports that are in addition to the standard, monthly data reports. Physicians are not paid for participating in the project, so the cost of operating this program is less than would be the case in the nonmilitary sector. All indirect costs (e.g., photocopying, travel) are also covered by the military, so do not contribute to the $2 million plus annual budget. The decision to expand the data base by enrolling more patients or adding another facility is based primarily on financial considerations. If additional money were available, more patients could be enrolled and CPDR could consider adding additional facilities.

Challenges, Recommendations, and Future Directions

One issue of interest is whether the CPDR data base could be merged into a national data base. Owing to the constraints of operating within the military structure, this would be extremely difficult if not impossible. CPDR staff anticipate that the military would not agree to share data with private-sector organizations. The main reason for this is the potential legal issues surrounding patient confidentiality and usage of the data, because the original patient consent for use of the information was limited to the objectives of CPDR. Combining the CPDR data with data from other data bases would require that each patient in the current data base give new written consent. There is concern that this consent process would lead to significant patient attrition.

A significant challenge to creating any outcomes data base, which was noted by the developers of CPDR, is the politics involved in meeting the needs and interests of the multiple participating organizations and sites. Success depends heavily on securing the cooperation and collaboration of all parties involved, and getting researchers, physicians, and hospitals to work together is time consuming, resource intensive, and requires commitment by all the players. Physicians are likely to need incentives to encourage their participation, such as data management and reporting tools that help them manage care for their patients and avoidance of redundant systems for capturing information.

All the facilities for the CPDR are located in large cities, and patients from small cities and rural areas are therefore not represented in the data base. It is conceivable that patients in these areas are different or that their care experiences are different. For example, military retirees might move to smaller towns and be less likely to receive care from one of the participating facilities. It is possible that these patients might therefore be older and have a different cancer profile, different treatment patterns, and different outcomes compared to those patients from the 11 major centers. It is unknown whether the care differs between participating and nonparticipating hospital centers and whether patients at nonparticipating centers experience worse outcomes. The data base may not be representative of all men nationally to the extent that military personnel are more physically fit than the general population of men with prostate cancer.

If the CPDR were to be replicated in the nonmilitary sector, CPDR estimates that the annual cost to develop and maintain such a data base would be three times as high or $6 million annually.

The CPDR data base provides one of the best examples of the organizational elements needed to develop and maintain a national data base on prostate cancer and outcomes, but this is partly a function of the unique characteristics of the military, which may not be replicable in the nonmilitary sector.

Prostate Disease Patient Outcomes Research Team

In 1989, the Agency for Health Care Policy and Research (AHCPR) funded the Patient Outcomes Research Teams (PORTs) to attempt to answer questions about the effectiveness and cost-effectiveness of available treatments for common clinical conditions (Freund et al., 1999). One of the PORTs funded by AHCPR addressed benign prostatic hyperplasia (BPH) (Wennberg et al., 1993). The project involved a group of researchers from Dartmouth, Massachusetts General Hospital, and the University of Massachusetts.

Each of the PORTs was obligated to conduct a formal literature review on what was known about the outcomes of treatment for the disease. The PORT projects were also to use readily available data—observational in nature—to advance the understanding of outcomes of care as applied to patients in everyday practice. The PORTs often used Medicare and Medicaid claims data, hospital cost report and discharge abstracts, and encounter data from health plans. The PORT approach stood in contrast to the traditional approach of conducting randomized clinical trials (RCTs) to answer questions regarding whether one treatment is more effective than another.

The PORT strategy for constructing an outcomes data base also contrasts with those previously described in this chapter. Rather than first collecting the data and then building the decision support tool, the prostate disease PORT built the decision aid first, followed by the prospective longitudinal data base to follow up patients according to their choice of treatment. This approach was designed to fill in gaps and to test specific hypotheses.

The team began by conducting a literature review and convening focus groups of patients to identify the outcomes of interest to patients. The research team then built a decision tree that included all of the outcomes relevant to patients, populating it with estimates (i.e., probabilities) of the chances that a given outcome will occur, according to patient subgroup if possible. The probability estimates were derived from an evidence-based review of the literature, analysis of existing data bases, and patient surveys to augment the data base with patient reports of outcomes (e.g., incidence of incontinence, impotence, disease recurrence). In some cases, the probability estimates for outcomes of interest were weak or missing.

Once the task of assigning probability estimates was completed, the team used this information to build a decision support tool to promote shared decision-making between physician and patient regarding choice of treatment. The decision aid took the best available information on outcomes estimates and presented prognostic information by subgroups of patients. The decision tool attempted to help patients make decisions that included outcome states for which, at the moment of decision, they would have had no direct experience. Where outcome information was weak or missing, the decision aid informed patients of the limits of scientific data.

The prostate disease PORT then built the longitudinal data base through systematic follow up of patients in clinical settings where the decision aids are routinely employed. The PORT approach differs from the RCT and the prostate cancer data bases described above in that the strategy for populating the probability estimates comes from people who have participated actively in the choice of treatment. In effect, the decision support tool is a mechanism for assigning patients to the treatments they prefer.

As noted in Chapter 1, Wennberg and colleagues (1993) propose an alternative strategy to RCTs for generating outcomes information, called the Preference Clinical Trial or PCT (i.e., patients choose among all treatments after being offered information about the risks and benefits of conventional and experimental treatments). The PCT approach (1) implements shared decision-making for all patients at a given center who are eligible for surgery, (2) helps patients come to a decision, (3) for those with preferences, enrolls them in the "preference arm" of the study, (4) for those who have no preference, offer a randomized clinical trial. All patients are followed in the same manner. This approach, observe the researchers, would provide an opportunity to examine differences in outcomes according to preference or randomized designs, and thus would provide information on external validity as well as information relevant to the question of the role patient expectation plays in determining health care outcomes.

When the BPH PORT was operational in the 1990s, the costs for conducting research to build the synthesized data base and decision support tools were $1 million per year.

Memorial Sloan Kettering Longitudinal Patient Data Base

This data base is resident in the hospital and tracks patients longitudinally to generate data to run medical statistical prediction models (i.e., nomograms). Partin nomograms (Partin et al., 1997) are statistical models that use patient clinical characteristics (i.e., PSA level, clinical stage, and Gleason score) to predict pathological stage for men with localized prostate cancer. This is important because as many as 50 percent of men undergoing radical prostatectomy were found to have extraprostatic disease at the time of surgery, rather than organ-confined disease. Patients undergoing radical prostatectomy for localized prostate cancer who have organ-confined disease demonstrate markedly improved biochemical disease-free survival compared with men who demonstrate extraprostatic disease (Pound et al., 1997). The authors in this study note that clinicians can use these nomograms when counseling individual patients regarding the probability of their tumor being at a specific pathological stage, so that they can make more informed treatment decisions.

At Memorial Sloan Kettering Cancer Center (MSKCC), clinicians have been tracking clinical outcomes for their own patients who receive radical prostatectomy, external beam radiation, and brachytherapy. Their statistical models or nomograms use PSA value, Gleason sum, and clinical stage to help predict biochemical freedom from recurrence for radical prostatectomy, external beam radiation, and brachytherapy. Only variables that were significant on multivariate analysis are included in the nomogram. These clinicians find that socioeconomic status and race factor out of outcome analysis for each stage and grade; these variables are related to diagnosis and time of diagnosis. The nomograms at this point do not incorporate any data on quality-of-life. The outcomes predicted by the nomograms reflect only those drawn from the experience of the physicians at Sloan Kettering.

In the future, the analyses will be used to predict clinical endpoints, such as metastasis-free survival, or to use additional pathology data, such as a percentage of cores positive and the individual Gleason grades. The current data base is static, meaning that the dataset is analyzed based on a data dump. The data base is currently being revamped with the long-term goal of making the nonogram output dynamic, or based on real-time routine data input. This will involve making the data base Web-based and not disclosing personal health information. The system will be used by other academic centers besides Sloan Kettering in the near future to validate the outcomes observed for the physicians at Sloan Kettering. At MSKCC, it will be used by the departments of urology and medicine. Estimates of the cost to produce these statistical modeling tools for surgery and brachytherapy are $120,000, which does not cover data entry or maintenance costs.

National Cancer Data Base

The American College of Surgeons' National Commission on Cancer (NCC) has established a National Cancer Data Base (NCDB), which is a nationwide oncology outcomes data base for over 1,500 hospitals in the United States. This NCDB is a partnership between the American College of Surgeons and the American Cancer Society to collect and report data on patterns of care and outcomes for all cancers. Annually, the NCDB issues a call for data to approximately 2,000 participating hospitals. The NCDB requests that hospitals voluntarily submit patient information (de-identified) to the national data base and requires hospitals to collect data items required by the Commission on Cancer (CoC). The CoC has constructed a list of specific data elements, data definitions, and coding instructions for the participating hospitals to follow (*Standards of the Commission on Cancer*, Volume II: *Registry Operations and Data Standards*). The NCDB, while not set up as a longitudinal tracking data base for use by physicians and patients, may provide a platform for recruiting hospitals and physicians across the United States to provide data on prostate cancer patients undergoing oncology treatment.

Prostate Cancer Research Institute

Although not specifically a data base used to track longitudinally men diagnosed with prostate cancer, the Prostate Cancer Research Institute (PCRI) is a unique resource for prostate cancer patients who are trying to gather information to make treatment decisions. PCRI was founded by medical oncologists with the goal of patient education to empower men to seek earlier diagnosis and to know the pros and cons of various treatment options. PCRI operates "Patient to Physician" (P2P) via the Internet, which is a moderated mailing list that permits patients to ask focused, clinical questions about prostate cancer. Patients receive timely responses from physician experts and are encouraged to discuss the information with their doctors. Through this special-interest discussion group, patients can see the responses to questions asked by other patients. This is an example of an informational resource for providing patients with prostate cancer medical information tailored to their unique circumstances, which can be used to engage in shared decision-making with their clinicians.

Summary

A number of data base efforts currently demonstrate the feasibility of securing the initial and ongoing participation of patients and physicians in the longitudinal monitoring of outcomes from prostate cancer treatment. These efforts have developed out of an interest in being able to understand the consequences of treatment and to guide future treatment decisions with respect to patient safety and the delivery of high-quality care. Table 1 summarizes the ability of current data base efforts to address the key questions of interest to patients and physicians to help guide treatment choices. As can be seen, there are still important gaps in the information desired as well as how the information is communicated to patients to assist with their decision-making.

None of the data bases reviewed fully realizes the People Like Me concept—one that allows patients, either directly or with their physicians, to create a subset of the data in ways personally relevant to them (by demographic and/or clinical characteristics) and to assess how outcomes of care compare and contrast based on the personal characteristics of the patient. None of the existing efforts has undertaken the step of drawing out the information learned regarding the different probabilities of experiencing different outcomes of interest to patients and creating a decision-support tool that patients can use to assess the risks and benefits of various treatment options. Of the existing data bases, PCOS may represent a viable platform for building a prototype People Like Me data base, because of its attempt to capture a nationally representative cross-section of the prostate cancer population and its focus on evaluating a broad range of patient outcomes.

Table 1: Can the Key Patient Questions be Addressed By Existing Data Bases?

Question	PCOS	SEER	CaPSURE	CPDR	Sloan Kettering
What are the side effects associated with surgery and how common are they?	Yes	No	Yes	Yes	No
What are the side effects of radiation therapy and how common are they?	Yes	No	Yes	Yes	No
What are the side effects of watchful waiting and how common are they?	Yes	No	Yes	Yes	No
What are the odds that I will be diagnosed with prostate cancer at 50? 60? 70? 80?	No	Yes	No	Yes	No
Does early initiation of treatment make a difference in clinical outcomes?	No, requires RCT	No	Can evaluate outcomes based on clinical characteristics impacted by stage migration and from date of diagnosis.	Yes	No
Does early initiation of treatment make a difference in functional outcomes?	No, requires RCT	No	Can provide information on health related quality-of-life (HRQOL) and function based on stage of disease and time from diagnosis and type of treatment.	Yes	No
What are the characteristics of patients who are choosing surgery?	Yes	Yes	Yes	Yes	Yes
What are the characteristics of patients who are choosing radiation?	Yes	Yes	Yes (data base does not represent radiation oncology patients)	Yes	Yes
What are the characteristics of patients who are choosing watchful waiting?	Yes	No	Yes	Yes	No

Table 1 - Continued

Question	PCOS	SEER	CaPSURE	CPDR	Sloan Kettering
If I get a side effect is there anything I can do? Is it permanent?	Survey asks about side effects. Long-term data analysis will answer question of permanency.	No	Addresses frequency of side effects and impact of impotence and other medications on outcome.	Not sure if data are collected.	No
Will herbal or supplemental therapies help me?	No. Survey asks if any taken, but does not specify type.	No	Can identify people using complementary and alternative medicine therapies.	Not sure if data are collected.	No
Does my diet matter?	No	No	No	Not sure if data are collected.	No
Does physical exercise make a difference?	No. Survey asks about limitations in activity.	No	No	Not sure if data are collected.	No
Is it okay if I drink alcohol?	No	No	No. Has information on smoking and alcohol use, not sufficient to determine a causal effect.	Not sure if data are collected.	No
Is it okay if I smoke?	No	No	No. Has information on smoking and alcohol use, not sufficient to determine a causal effect.	Not sure if data are collected.	No

Strategy for Constructing a National Prostate Cancer Outcomes Data Base

To create a blueprint for constructing a national prostate cancer outcomes data base, we define key design aspects of the data base to fully actualize the People Like Me concept. As a caveat, the strategy outlined below will require refinement based on various assumptions about how the data base should be designed and what it should include. For example, we are assuming that data collection commences when a patient has a positive diagnosis of prostate cancer. An alternative, not discussed here, is to commence data collection with PSA screening so as to track patients prior to becoming active cancer cases; however, one concern with this strategy is the potential for bias because not all men elect to undergo screening. Consequently, finding the appropriate at-risk population to participate would be difficult.

Content of the Data Base

The exact content of the data base needs to be determined by the goals of the data base and specific set of questions that it is designed to address. While we have attempted to identify the key questions of interest through our consultations with clinicians and patient advocates, we believe more work is required to refine the list of questions and to achieve consensus by clinicians, researchers, and patients on the outcomes that will be assessed and reported to various audiences. The contents of the data base should not be static and the data base will have to be designed to accommodate and reflect any changes in the treatments available and/or disease course over time. This may require the addition and subtraction of variables as well as changing data definitions. In our discussions with staff from various data base endeavors, it was noted that the data elements contained in the data base require continual review and updating—an important aspect of the ongoing maintenance of any data base effort.

At a minimum, data should be collected on all standard therapeutic options including watchful waiting, radical prostatectomy (surgery to remove the prostate), brachytherapy (radioactive seed implantation), external beam radiation, orchiectomy (removal of the testes), and androgen deprivation. Treatment data need to be detailed to understand the exact type of treatment provided to the patient (e.g., whether treatment involved conventional external beam or conformal external beam radiation). Given significant interest among patients in alternative therapies and virtually no studies to examine outcomes, the People Like Me data base may provide an opportunity to collect information on alternative treatments (either alone or in combination with standard treatments) and to assess outcomes. Should a decision be made to include alternative treatments, substantial effort will need to be applied to defining these treatments so that data can be collected in a standardized way. No existing data structure on alternative treatments has been designed or tested that is ready for immediate application, so considerable work will be required to address this issue.

In addition to the treatment variables, the data base should capture

- contact information for the patient—name, address, phone, e-mail address, consent
- contact information for the provider—name, address, phone, e-mail address
- dates of treatment
- demographic/patient information—age, life expectancy, family history of prostate cancer, history of other cancer, insurance coverage, education,

income, race/ethnicity, primary language spoken, satisfaction with treatment

- clinical information—pretreatment clinical stage (digital rectal exam), pretreatment Gleason score, pretreatment total PSA, comorbidities, use of hormone therapy, pretreatment urinary, sexual, and bowel function, list of visits and details for each visit, hospitalization information, biopsy, medications, pathology, pre- and posttreatment physical, mental and social functioning, posttreatment Gleason scores and PSA
- outcome information—survival (one, five, 10 year), fatigue, posttreatment physical, mental and social functioning, posttreatment urinary, sexual, and bowel function
- provider characteristics (physician and hospital)—board certification, specialty, annual volume of procedures, teaching versus community hospital, and other proxy variables of differences in the care a patient might receive (e.g., urban versus rural).

Sources of Data

Information to populate the data base will need to come from both clinicians and patients. Information such as lab values, pathology reports, imaging, staging of disease, clinical description of the tumor, description of the treatment, complications, functional status, intermediate and long-term outcomes, and characteristics of the physician (e.g., volume of procedures, training) can be compiled from the physician—preferably from clinical records. Patients should not be asked to provide information about treatments and staging, for which they may have poor recall. Patients can provide information on their functional status (physical, mental, and social) and intermediate and long-term outcomes. To facilitate the buy-in of physicians to provide information on a sustained basis, efforts would need to be made to avoid creating redundancies in record-keeping; this could be achieved if the data base served a record-keeping function for their practice.

Approaches to Obtaining Data

The differing methods of recruitment used by existing data bases have different implications for the cost of the project and potential for bias. One strategy is to mimic the PCOS and start by identifying a sample of patients. PCOS draws a sample of patients from the SEER cancer registry data base, which by design is national in scope and seeks to capture a representative sample of cancer patients. Following a design such as PCOS offers the advantage of being able to identify and recruit a representative sample of patients into the data base. The downside of this approach is that physicians are not directly engaged to work with patients to encourage and reinforce participation, so response rates to surveys are likely to be lower. It also potentially involves engaging a larger number of clinical practice sites from which to collect clinical data on patients because this approach does not require recruiting all prostate cancer patients within a given physician's practice. Consequently, the fixed costs are likely to be higher in this model if only a small number of patients in any single provider's practice are part of the data base.

An alternative approach is to sample providers first—both oncologists and urologists—and then to recruit patients from the selected providers. This is a cluster-sample strategy, and the process might first select cities and some rural areas that represent a broad cross-section of patient and clinical practice sites nationally, then sample providers within those geographic areas, and finally take either some or all patients for each provider in the sample. This strategy has the advantages of engaging providers to serve as agents to help in recruitment of patients and may achieve cost economies by gathering multiple patients and their data from each practice site chosen for inclusion in the study. Unlike the provider-focused recruitment efforts used in some of the existing data bases, which were based on convenience samples, we recommend that the recruitment strategy be based on a random or stratified sample of providers who would represent the range of providers that patients with prostate cancer would likely see for treating their cancer. The universe of radiation oncologists and urologists could potentially be identified using Medicare data files.

In any sampling strategy to obtain the data, it will likely be necessary to fill holes in the sample—for instance, for the poor and uninsured or underinsured who may not receive care from the same type of providers identified in the core sample.

Recruitment of and Participation by Patients and Providers

Given the positive response among prostate cancer patients at the consultation meetings, it is likely that initial patient participation would be high, provided that the purpose of the data collection was explained, that patients understand that this information would help others with prostate cancer, that the entity compiling the information could be "trusted," and that patient privacy and confidentiality is protected. Most of the data bases had relatively high rates of initial participation by patients, and those with the highest rates appeared to rely on face-to-face contact with the patient through physician-led recruiting. In PCOS, which relied upon contacting patients via mail or phone interview, response rates to the first request for data were 62 percent of the sampled population.

The greater challenge is ensuring sustained patient participation. Patient attrition was less than 1 percent in the military data base, which involves intensive patient follow up, 5 percent annually in CaPSURE, and 17 percent in the PCOS effort (24-month follow up survey). Some attrition is to be expected because patients die and others view themselves as disease free or "cured" five years after treatment. Engaging in frequent contact with patients appears to improve the likelihood of sustained participation, and most data bases seek to provide incentives to patients to sustain their interest, such as sending them newsletters on prostate cancer.

Physician participation rates were 100 percent in the military data base and 99 percent in the medical abstraction component of the PCOS study. The CaPSURE data base effort also was quite successful in recruiting physician sites, and was limited more by the availability of financial resources to support all sites expressing interest in participating.

Frequency of Data Collection

Once the patient is diagnosed with prostate cancer, baseline data collection should commence prior to any treatment (i.e., pretreatment functioning and clinical factors such as stage of disease, PSA, Gleason score, comorbidities). Clinical data are then collected again at time of treatment and follow up visits. In other studies, the frequency of subsequent data collection to evaluate patient functioning—as reported directly by patients—generally occurs at 6 months, 12 months, 18 - 24 months, and then annually thereafter. More-frequent data collection was found to be expensive and burdensome to the patient, and did not produce additional information of value in predicting outcomes.

Sponsorship

Sponsorship refers to financial as well as organizational support for the data base project. It is a critical factor in securing the participation of patients and providers. Patients indicated that they view an organization such as the American Cancer Society as a respected and trusted source of patient information and thus a good candidate for sponsoring a data base. Patients also noted that the National Cancer Institute, a federal agency, was a trusted source of information on prostate cancer, and they would view this entity as a credible sponsor. The key concern expressed by patients is that they did not want the sponsor to be an organization that would have access to and share their personal data or gain financially from having access to their data, such as pharmaceutical companies.

The nature of the data collection and products to be derived from the People Like Me prostate cancer data base speak to engaging multiple organizations in sponsoring the effort—including patient advocacy groups like the American Cancer Society Man-to-

Man support groups, Us-Too International, Cap Cure, and the National Prostate Cancer Coalition, research entities such as the National Cancer Institute (both for its research expertise and communications to patients), the American College of Surgeons' National Commission on Cancer, the Radiation Therapy Oncology Group, and urology and oncology physician organizations such as the American Urological Association and the American Society for Therapeutic Radiation and Oncology. These players should be engaged in helping to define the effort, providing support for patient and provider participation, and potentially as a funding source. A consortium of organizations such as these, in concert with one or more foundations, could potentially provide start-up funds to design and operationalize the data base. Foundations typically support "start-up" efforts, so the project would need to identify long-term financial sponsors to sustain the effort—such as government agencies and/or patient support groups.

Constructing the Information Tool

Once the data are compiled for the purposes of determining whether patients experience differences in outcomes from treatment, the next challenge is packaging the information in a way that is usable for consumers and physicians. The approach to organizing and displaying the information needs to be given considerable thought and testing, because the cognitive psychology and decision-making sciences research finds that the way information is framed and the complexity of the data display affect whether the information is used to make decisions and what choices are made (Slovic, 1995; Hibbard et al., 2002). How the material is presented (e.g., mortality versus survival) can influence individual decisions about which treatment to choose; consequently, it is important that the direction and the extent of the influence of the display formats be known and defensible. A key responsibility of the information producer is to produce information that can be used by consumers for choice but will not influence their decision-making in unintended ways. This will require mocking up various prototypes of the decision tool and testing them with patients for design influences—in addition to standard cognitive testing for comprehension and usability. Developers of the consumer information platform will also need to be sensitive to the presentation of complex information for audiences with varying levels of literacy.

As use of the Internet increases and given the structure of Web-based platforms for disseminating information—which allow for easier and cheaper approaches to tailoring information to individual users—the decision aid tool derived from the People Like Me national data base would likely be a computer-based platform. A computer-assisted decision tool can potentially help with the challenge consumers face in processing and weighing various factors to make a choice—especially if the information is tailored to their own situation. While a computer platform may work for a majority of users, the developers will need to better understand what avenues and preferences consumers have for accessing the information (e.g., print materials, video tapes), because not all patients and their families will have access to the Internet.

The time it takes to develop a computer-aided decision tool will need to be factored into the overall project timeline; this product by itself will likely take two to three years to develop.

Cost Analysis

In our review of existing data bases, we asked the staff within each of the projects to define the costs they incurred to develop and operate their data bases on an ongoing basis. While several of the projects were willing to share information about staffing and costs, often these estimates were not of sufficient detail to allow us to construct detailed cost estimates. At best, the cost and staffing figures they did provide give a sense of the magnitude of resource investment that would be required. For several of the projects or for components within projects, we could not obtain cost data because those figures were considered proprietary.

The CaPSURE data base, which tracks 8,100 patients and seeks to add approximately 1,500 new enrollees each year, has a budget of $3.5 million to cover 20 staff at UCSF. The budget covers recruitment of sites, data collection, data cleaning, programming and analysis, research support, and physician incentive payments ($150/patient initially and $100/patient annually thereafter). This figure does not include the costs for staff at the pharmaceutical firm and the third party software vendor that hosts the data collection and reporting tool. Using the $3.5 million estimate, the annual cost per patient is roughly $432.

The PCOS data base has spent between $7 and $10 million over the last eight years (1994 - 2002) to track approximately 3,500 patients, for an average annual cost per patient of $286 (if one assumes that approximately $1 million per year is spent). This budget covers four staff located at the National Cancer Institute and an unknown number of people working with the six SEER registries.

The CPDR data base is funded at $2 million annually and receives additional annual grant support of between $500,000 to $1 million to track 16,000 patients. This works out to an average annual cost of $188 per patient (if one assumes $3 million per year as the budget). This figure covers the CPDR staff and 18 data managers' salaries. However, it is important to note that this level of funding does not support the full cost of operating the program. All indirect costs (photocopying, office space, travel, phone) are covered by the military, and physicians are prohibited from receiving incentive payments to participate. If all of these costs were included, the cost of operating the program would be much higher. CPDR estimates that to replicate its data base in the nonmilitary sector would cost approximately $6 million annually.

Final cost estimates will be a function of the size of the patient and physician population tracked, the scope of the effort (number of variables, number of unique sites, amount of data collection, and method of data collection), and whether incentive payments are required to enhance participation. In addition, if a patient-based approach to recruitment is pursued, it may be more costly to implement because of the need to go to many more physician and hospital sites (i.e., the economy of getting all patients at any given physician site is lost and now only a single patient may be enrolled for any given provider).

It should also be emphasized that the cost estimates listed above do not reflect what the actual costs of implementing a People Like Me data base would be, because none of these efforts captures the costs of taking information from the data base and organizing, packaging, and disseminating it to patients and providers throughout the United States. It could cost several million dollars to develop a consumer decision aid; hundreds of thousands of dollars annually to maintain the decision-support tool; and several million more to maintain and disseminate the information. As a result, building a fully functional large-scale data collection system and patient-provider decision support tool could require annual funding in the range of $5 to $10 million.

A Staged Approach to Building a National Outcomes Data Base

Establishing the data base will be a multiyear, complex undertaking. Interim steps can be taken to facilitate data base development and also provide useful information to consumers until such time that a national data base is fully up and running and producing information to inform treatment decisions. First steps should include working with physicians and patients to refine the set of questions and specify which clinical and demographic factors are known to be important in influencing the outcomes (i.e., the stratifying variables such as PSA level or Gleason score).

Those who currently operate data bases felt it would be critical to convene a group that would develop a consensus on what outcomes information could or should be released to patients and to clearly define these measures. Another interim step would be to take the set of questions and determine which questions existing data collection efforts or research initiatives have already provided or could provide answers to with additional data mining, and to grade the strength of the evidence. This evaluation would seek to address the questions using the People Like Me concept, by attempting to produce outcomes results by key patient characteristics (age, Gleason score, PSA, comorbidities). In the process of putting existing data bases to the People Like Me test, we could learn where the information holes are and define appropriate strategies for filling those holes—whether it be a national longitudinal data base or a randomized controlled trial. From the review of the existing data, several researchers thought that information already exists that could be packaged and disseminated to patients to aid them with making treatment choices.

Table 2 outlines the set of steps required to develop a national outcomes data base and the approximate length of time required to accomplish each step. As part of the development process, we include a step focused on exploring opportunities for culling information from existing data sources as a means to flesh out the gaps in the knowledge and data collection processes. However, even if existing data sources provide some of the desired information, there remains the need to invest in analyzing, organizing, and presenting the information in ways that are relevant to patients and that can be used and understood by patients for the purposes of evaluating treatment options. As Table 2 shows, it would take approximately four to five years to fully design and implement the data collection process and to disseminate information to patients.

Table 2: Timeline and Key Milestones for Developing Data Base

Key Milestones	Timeline
I. Planning Stage	
Define specific purpose of data base, who will use information, and how that information will be disseminated.	Months 1 - 3
Identify key constituencies to be collaborators in the project (e.g., American Cancer Society, National Cancer Institute, prostate cancer patient advocacy groups, urologists and radiation oncologists). Solicit feedback, input, and support from appropriate patient and provider constituency groups; begin to lay ground work for working collaboratively with these patient and provider groups to promote the benefits of participating in the data base and securing the commitment of physicians and patients to supply data. Form advisory panel to provide policy and technical guidance on the development of the data base.	Months 1 - 6
Refine the set of questions the data base will seek to answer and engage patients, clinicians, and researchers in a consensus development exercise to specify and define the set of outcome measures that will be measured and reported out to patients and physicians.	Months 1 - 12
Define and gain consensus from the patient, clinical, and research community on the set of stratifying variables (covariates) that are predictive factors in determining outcomes and that patients will be able to use to query the data base to get answers for People Like Me. Patients with prostate cancer should be asked to specify how they would like to query the data.	Months 1 - 12

Table 2 – Continued

Key Milestones	Timeline
Review existing data collection efforts and the published literature from these studies/project to determine which questions can be answered already by the relevant People Like Me subsetting variables. Grade the level of evidence contained in the research studies. Identify where the gaps remain that a new data base effort could fill. Seek to construct a collaborative pooling of data across data collection efforts so as to be able to conduct cross-site analyses, and to standardize data definitions, data collection tools, and outcomes of interest.	Months 1 - 18
Define the mechanisms for collecting the data (survey, administrative data, chart abstraction).	Months 12 - 24
Define the sampling method for selecting physicians and patients.	Months 12 - 18
Take the "key questions" to be addressed by the data base and define the set of data elements required and operationalize the definitions. Identify the data source and frequency of collection for each element. Determine whether new data collection tools are required or whether existing tools can be modified.	Months 12 - 24
Develop new data collection tools (if necessary).	Months 12 - 24
Prepare training materials (training manual, data code book).	Months 18 - 24
Design a pilot test of the data collection tools and processing protocols.	Months 18 - 24
II. Pilot Stage	
Identify a small number of practice sites (<=5) to pilot test the data collection methodology.	Months 18 - 24
Train pilot site personnel on data collection methods.	Months 24 - 25
Commence data collection in pilot sites.	Months 25 - 36
Interview staff at each of the practice sites to identify what worked and did not work during "implementation."	Months 30 - 36
Review data that are submitted during pilot phase to assess completeness, consistency, and accuracy.	Months 26 - 36
Revise data collection tools and procedures.	Months 36 - 37
III. Full-Scale Implementation of Data Collection	
Expand data collection to more practice sites—recruit providers and patients into the study.	Months 38 - 54
Conduct training of personnel in each site on the data collection.	Months 38 - 54
Begin collecting data; technical assistance to sites.	Months 39 +
Ongoing recruitment of sites, training, data collection.	Months 40 +
IV. Data Analysis	
Data processing protocols—data cleaning, auditing, analysis.	Months 39 +
Organize results for distribution to providers and patients.	Months 48 +

Table 2 – Continued

Key Milestones	Timeline
V. Development of Information/Decision Support Tool	
Meet with patient representatives to define the content of the information resource and how it should be communicated.	Months 12 - 15
Meet with physician representatives to define the information they would like to see presented for use by physicians to assist with making treatment decisions.	Months 15 - 18
Review the cognitive literature on consumer/patient decision-making to guide the design of the information resource.	Months 15 - 20
Develop a mock-up of a prototype decision support tool for review by patients and physicians.	Months 20 - 26
Conduct testing with patients/consumers for design influences (e.g., framing, use of language), comprehension, and usability.	Months 26 - 30
Build consumer information tool.	Months 36 - 48
VI. Dissemination/Public Awareness	
Build awareness among the patient and provider community that a tool is available to assist with making treatment decisions (public education campaign).	Months 48 - 56

Feasibility Considerations: Issues That Need to be Addressed in Building a National Prostate Cancer Outcomes Data Base

Bias in the Sample of Patients

Observational data bases, properly designed, should be inclusive of all patients who have the condition and receive treatment, even if it is watchful waiting. How physicians and patients are recruited into the longitudinal tracking effort will influence the degree to which one can make outcome predictions that are valid and generalizable to the broad population of prostate cancer patients. The results of most existing prostate cancer data collection efforts may be biased or of limited generalizability because they only include patients who are on specific treatment protocols, who are from medical centers with selected characteristics, or who are in certain age groups. For the People Like Me outcomes data base that would be used by patients and providers to compare treatment options, the strategy for recruiting and including patients in the data base should allow for the collection of data from patients and physicians that represents the full patient population and set of treatment options (surgery, radiation, hormone, watchful waiting). Doing so will minimize the potential for bias in the results.

The initial sampling or recruitment strategy—if provider based—should focus on getting a broad mix of providers (e.g., urologists, radiation oncologists, and primary care providers) and ensuring the highest possible patient participation in each of those sites.

A patient-based recruitment strategy, depending on the level of response rates achieved, runs the risk of nonrespondent bias if response rates are low. Consequently, efforts (i.e., aggressive follow up, provision of incentives) should be made to maximize response rates and also to assess the degree to which bias may be present. One approach is to assess whether the sample of participants is different from nonparticipants, which requires the collection of a small number of descriptive data elements on all potential participants (i.e., those invited to participate). Many of the existing data base efforts reviewed for this report do attempt to collect a minimum set of data elements on all persons invited to join the data base.

Size of the Patient Sample Needed to Develop an Outcomes Data Base

The sample size required for an outcomes data base is mainly a function of the number of People Like Me patient characteristics (e.g., age, race/ethnicity, stage of disease) or subsetting variables desired that are related to the outcomes of interest. In a study of prostate cancer outcomes by Litwin et al. (2000), the authors identify a handful of clinical covariates that might be important covariates associated with the various prostate cancer outcomes. These variables include patient age, patient life expectancy, pretreatment total PSA, clinical stage, Gleason grade, family history of prostate cancer, history of other cancer, and comorbidity indicators. Additional covariates would likely include treatment type, the use of hormone therapy, insurance coverage, race/ethnicity, education, and income. As more subsetting variables are added to allow patients and their physicians to tailor the output in a way unique to the individual patient, more patients must be tracked to ensure adequate sample sizes in each analytic cell (e.g., an analytic cell could be defined by a specific age range of the patient, race/ethnicity, and treatment type).

It is more difficult to detect differences among small subgroups in the population than among larger groups. Estimates for small subgroups of patients will have larger standard errors (i.e., more uncertainty in the estimate). Consequently, it may be worth considering, for certain variables such as age, displaying information across a range (e.g., ages 50 - 60) to address the problem of small sample sizes. Clinicians and patients would need to jointly determine acceptable and biologically appropriate ranges for variables that would represent aggregations, as well as the subsetting variables and outcomes of interest.

Because most patients would like information to be closely tailored to their own experience, it will be necessary to collect data on a large number of people across a diversity of patients. This desire will need to be balanced with cost issues associated with tracking more individuals and the prevalence of selected outcomes. For example, to study rare treatment combinations or rare outcomes, it would be essential to get data on all patients (as in a census or registry like the End Stage Renal Disease program)—something that would be more difficult and costly than sampling patients.

To estimate the size of the sample needed to develop an outcomes data base requires making certain assumptions. For the calculations below, we have assumed that the outcomes data base will be used for regression analyses that are multivariate in nature. This includes contrasts between two groups (or t-tests) as a special case. However, it excludes reducing the data by conditioning on certain variables or strata and then contrasting outcomes within the subset of the data.

We have also assumed that, in most cases, higher-order interactions beyond two-level interactions are not significant or policy relevant (i.e., for large data sets interaction terms between two variables may be statistically significant but the coefficients are too small to matter in practice). Because of the normal approximation to the binomial distribution we can use power calculations based on the normal distribution with variance 0.5. Table 3 shows sample sizes needed under various scenarios. We have computed the estimates as a function of the smallest detectable difference that one would expect to observe between outcomes of interest (e.g., a 20-percentage-point difference in mortality) and the possible presence of two-level interactions. Calculations are based on a significance level of $\alpha = 0.05$ and 80 percent power to detect the effect. The calculations represent the worst-case situation where the probability is $p_1 = 0.5$.

Table 3: Sample Size for Each Category

Number of patients for each cell created by subsetting	Smallest detectable difference in outcomes (percentage point)	Presence of two-level interaction effects
99	20	No
197	20	Yes
175	15	No
349	15	Yes
393	10	No
785	10	Yes
1,570	5	No
3,139	5	Yes

If the subsetting variable or covariate—such as race—contains more than two levels, the sample size shown in Table 3 above is required for each of the levels. If the covariate is continuous these calculations still hold and can be considered conservative. If the outcome variable is continuous, the approach is still valid, but Table 3 does not apply because it assumes a percentage for the smallest detectable difference. Instead, an estimate of mean and variance of the outcome variable is needed to do the power calculations.

To help illustrate the implications of Table 3, we estimate the required number of patients for the following data base example. Let's say we are interested in evaluating differences in five-year survival rates for different forms of treatment on the following patient characteristics (variables with the number of "levels" shown in parentheses behind each): age (continuous), pretreatment PSA (continuous), clinical stage (four levels), Gleason grade (continuous), comorbidities (three levels), race/ethnicity (five levels), education (three levels), and insurance coverage (three levels). Assuming that the data base is perfectly balanced across covariates and that we are not throwing away information by subsetting (i.e., we are producing estimates using regression analysis that uses all of the information available), then we would take our largest number of levels—in this case five for race/ethnicity—and multiply by the "number of patients for each cell" shown in Table 3. Thus, for a 10-percentage point difference in five-year survival and no interaction effects (393 patients per cell), we would minimally need 1,965 patients. For a five-percentage point difference in outcome with no interactions (1,570 patients per cell), we would need 7,850 patients. If the variable is not balanced, more patients would be required.

Table 3 represents a worst-case scenario where the probabilities of interest are around 0.5. Table 4 considers several small probabilities explicitly, and the resulting sample sizes are much smaller (roughly one-third to one-half the previous sample sizes). Table 4 stems from ordinary power calculations based on a binomial distribution. Interactions were not considered. Calculations are based on a significance level of $\alpha = 0.05$ and 80-percent power to detect an effect.

Table 4: Sample Size for Each Category as a Function of Various Smaller Probabilities

Number of patients for each subsetting variable	p1	p2	Smallest detectable difference (percentage point)
59	0.05	0.25	20
88	0.05	0.20	15
160	0.05	0.15	10
474	0.05	0.10	5

We provide another example to illustrate the sample size calculations. In prostate cancer, one of the outcome variables of interest is presence or absence of hospitalization, medical or surgical treatment for cystitis, proctitis, hematuria, or rectal bleeding. Each of these is a dichotomous variable. Suppose we determine that the covariates to be used in the regression analysis are patient has/does not have insurance, pretreatment total PSA, and clinical stage. Further suppose that we are interested in all two-level interactions and that three-level interactions are negligible.

To detect a difference in the outcome variable of 10 percentage points (e.g. 50 percent versus 60 percent) under the usual power and significance assumptions, we would require 785 patients in each variable category. Thus, there need to be 785 patients with insurance and 785 patients without insurance. There also needs to be 2 x 785 patients whose PSA score roughly covers the range of interest (i.e., is not concentrated in a small area of the range). If the data base is perfectly balanced across all covariates this can be accomplished with 2 x 785 = 1,570 patients. In practice, the number will be somewhat larger because the data base is unlikely to be perfectly balanced across all categories. If we consider more than three explanatory variables, the sample size requirement does not change. However, the more variables there are, the more likely it is that some categories do not have 785 patients. Since the same number of patients is needed for each category the sample will tend to be larger.

Some variables like race have more than two levels. The number of patients required, as determined from Table 3, needs to be available from each level within the variable category (e.g., for race, 785 whites, 785 African-American, 785 Asian, and so forth). Suppose it is known that African-Americans are difficult to recruit and that the data base may only successfully recruit 200. Based on Table 3, a sample of 200 African-American patients means that we would only be able to detect a difference of 20 percentage points for outcomes with interaction effects and a difference of (at least) 15 percentage points for main effects.

Sample size calculations always presume that the sample is drawn at random. Outcome data bases are generally not random because it is highly impractical and very costly to sample patients at random. To do so would require the existence of a national registry of patients. In theory, the lack of randomness limits statistical inferences that can be drawn from the sample. The lack of randomness is somewhat alleviated by ensuring that the sample is representative with respect to the relevant variables (e.g., all treatments, all treatment settings, and types of providers). Because the People Like Me subsetting approach explicitly considers important variables as covariates, it increases the likelihood of having a group of patients that is representative of the population of interest.

Throughout the sample size calculations shown thus far, we have assumed that the outcome variable is dichotomous (e.g., yes or no). If the outcome is continuous, the sample size needed will be substantially lower. This implies that the easiest way to increase power in analysis is to avoid creating discrete variables (either outcomes or predictors) wherever possible. For example, instead of collecting information on whether or not the patient survived until five years after a treatment (yes or no), it would be preferable to record the length of survival and conduct a survival analysis.

The sample sizes proposed in Table 3 are considered to be conservative. Throughout, we have assumed that we are trying to detect a difference of 0.5 versus an alternate value. This is conservative because, for example, it is much easier to detect 0.05 versus 0.1 than 0.5 versus 0.55. Therefore, the sample sizes displayed in Table 4 are much smaller.

The "curse of dimensionality" refers to the following phenomenon: the more variables that are considered simultaneously, the sparser the data appear. This "curse" applies to the following situation: If I wish to understand the outcome under different treatment alternatives for "people who are exactly like me" (i.e., for people who match my characteristics on all covariates), the number of people I am comparing to will be very small. The ability to draw conclusion on such a subgroup will be limited. A regression approach circumvents the curse of dimensionality by making use of the assumption that no higher-order interactions are relevant. This holds true in most practical situations.

As noted above, the desired patient sample size is dependent on whether one wishes to estimate interaction terms (to account for nonlinearities in the data) with sufficient power. The sample size recommendations accommodate both multivariate and univariate analyses. We do not accommodate within-strata analyses. (Note: A stratified or univariate display of the data may be misleading to patients because the outcomes represented do not take into account [or control for] other variables that may be important factors in determining the outcome. For example, looking at outcome results by age alone will miss the effect that clinical stage of the cancer has on predicting the outcome of interest, such as likelihood of survival.)

Outcomes to Be Measured

At the outset of the project, it will be critical to specify the key outcomes (e.g., survival, functioning, complications) that should be tracked. The process will benefit from soliciting input from and working toward consensus with the patient and clinical community that the specified outcomes are in fact the relevant endpoints of interest to the end users of the data base. Once the outcome measures are agreed to, additional work will be required to clearly define the measures (creating operational definitions) for the purposes of uniform data collection. For example, the measure would need to define the starting point (baseline could be from diagnosis or treatment) and the end point (e.g., in-hospital mortality, 30-day mortality, five-year mortality).

Throughout the design and ongoing operation of the data base, it will be necessary to solicit clinical input into what variables are being collected, how are they defined, and what role they play in analysis (are they predictors, are they descriptive). As occurs with any data collection effort, the data base will evolve over time—both its contents and its functions. Therefore, it will be important to seek ongoing feedback from data entry personnel in clinical practices and hospitals, clinicians, researchers, and patients to improve the data and the data base quality.

Data Base Architecture

One piece of feedback received from the existing data base projects was the need to store "raw" values to ensure flexibility to derive variables for various analyses. Because key variable definitions may change over time (e.g., the determination of clinical staging), having access to the raw data elements used to derive variables allows flexibility over time to use information collected in earlier time periods for analyses as definitions change. In examining all data elements, it will be important to determine which can be broken down into more granular elements and to be sure to track information at this level. A relational data base architecture will likely be most useful to allow the tracking of many different pieces of information that can be linked.

Data Quality

One of the areas that will affect the ability to produce reliable and valid outcome results is the underlying quality of the data supplied by clinicians, hospitals, and patients. As always, there is a risk of variation in how data are captured across sites that has nothing to do with real variation in patients, their care, or their outcomes. An important step in reducing variation is to have clearly defined and agreed-to variables and definitions for those variables. Other strategies to reduce variation in coding across sites is to have standardized data collection instruments and to engage staff from the sites providing the data in regular training sessions. However, despite these efforts, the project staff operating the data base will need to develop programs (i.e., data quality reports looking for out-of-range values and inconsistent information, occurrences of values for data elements that are well outside the average observed across all institutions) and maintain oversight to catch and correct problems with coding. These efforts can be reinforced with periodic audits of data being submitted by providers to verify the accuracy of data submissions. Auditing can be a costly activity because it usually involves going to a practice site and abstracting information from a clinical record. Audits can be designed to be cost-effective by focusing on a limited number of data elements (e.g., those that are most important), a limited number of sites each year, and being purposeful in selecting sites for audit (e.g., those that appear to have the most difficulty with coding or seem to have statistically better or worse performance results).

Data Output

There will likely be multiple end users of the data, including researchers, clinicians, and—most important—patients. Supporting the needs of the various end users will require understanding what information they would like to have and how they propose to manipulate the information. Patients might be given some flexibility to customize their searches based on a handful of clinical and demographic characteristics, whereas clinicians and research staff might be provided broader access to de-identified information for running analyses. Customization of output allows for different uses of the information by end users, but it is also more expensive to maintain. For patients in particular, little work has been done on how to develop an effective user interface for presenting outcomes information. Developing the interface will require an evaluation of alternative modes for efficient presentation of complex data to individuals with diverse information needs and preferences for involvement with treatment decisions.

Protection of Confidential Information and Patient Privacy

Any time someone gives personal information to someone else, maintaining the confidentiality of that information and ensuring patient privacy is a key concern. For the purposes of creating a longitudinal outcomes data base on prostate cancer, we would need to collect contact information on both the patient and the provider (including name, address, and possibly telephone number) for follow up data collection (both clinical and survey information). To gain the cooperation of patients and providers (and their affiliated institutions), it will be necessary to develop a plan to protect human subjects and have a policy for data safeguarding that is reviewed and approved by an Institutional Review Board.

Each patient would need to be assigned a research ID number when he completes the initial questionnaire. This way, information regarding functional status and outcomes can be kept separate from contact information, ensuring that people accessing the data base cannot obtain contact information for contributors. Patients must be assured that all data will remain confidential and that others will only be able to access data in aggregate form. Prior to the collection of any data, a procedure would be required to ensure that patient and physician privacy concerns are addressed.

CHAPTER 5:
OSTEOARTHRITIS DATA BASE FEASIBILITY ASSESSMENT

Background

Osteoarthritis in hips or knees, a chronic health condition, is the leading cause of disability among elderly Americans. As the elderly population continues to grow in the United States, the number of osteoarthritis cases is expected to increase. The CDC estimates that more than 60 million Americans will have the disease by 2050 and that the cost of treatment will exceed $65 billion, including medical treatment and lost productivity.

Treatments for osteoarthritis include diet, exercise, pharmacotherapy, surgery, and various holistic approaches. There is no cure for osteoarthritis. Treatments for osteoarthritis help slow the progression of the disease, ease pain, and increase patient function. Most patients have the disease for decades and thus are likely to face decisions about treatment strategies over the course of their lives. Although the efficacy of many osteoarthritis medications has been tested individually in clinical trials, there are no studies that compare and contrast differences in outcomes that different patients experience using alternative medications. It is a significant challenge to track the outcomes of the range of medication treatment combinations over the course of an arthritis patient's life given the number of possible medications a person could take in a lifetime and the sequence of those drugs.

Given the large number of Americans affected by osteoarthritis and the multitude of treatment options, osteoarthritis was considered a good candidate for investigating the need for and feasibility of establishing an outcomes data base. The assessment consisted of identifying a set of questions a data base could answer (Appendix B), engaging providers and patients in a discussion of the utility of the data base concept and issues related to the feasibility of collecting and organizing data that could be used by patients and their physicians, and examining existing data bases that are collecting outcomes information for osteoarthritis.

Consultative Meetings with Arthritis Patients and Provider Representatives

To assess the feasibility of creating a data base that would give patients and their physicians information on how arthritis treatments might affect them personally based on outcomes of treatment from other patients like them, we held two consultative meetings with patients and providers. The first meeting took place March 13, 2002 at the

AHRQ offices in Rockville, MD. At this meeting, attendees were primarily health care providers and researchers, including some who had worked with existing arthritis outcomes data bases (see Appendix D). The second meeting was held on June 19, 2002 at RAND in Santa Monica, CA and the attendees were all osteoarthritis patients who resided in the Los Angeles area.

The original intent of our first meeting was to bring together a range of providers and representatives of patient advocacy organizations to explore the feasibility of creating an outcomes data base on osteoarthritis treatments. However, because the Arthritis Foundation (AF) was the only patient advocacy group dedicated to the issues of interest, it was the sole "patient representative" at the first meeting. Given a desire for greater input by patients in our feasibility assessment, we decided to hold a second consultative meeting. For the second meeting, we recruited nine osteoarthritis patients from rheumatologists in the Los Angeles area to explore the set of questions. Because the focus of the project was on producing information that would be useful for patients, we felt the second meeting was essential to ensure we had identified patients' perspectives on these issues. During the two consultative meetings, we explored a wide range of potential questions that the data base could be designed to answer, and these draft questions are found in Appendix B.

We had originally selected arthritis as the condition of interest. However, arthritis is actually a collection of about 100 different diseases with different etiologies and treatments. To make the provider panel discussions more manageable, we focused on the two most common forms of arthritis—rheumatoid arthritis and osteoarthritis. The provider panel concluded that an outcomes data base could not combine these two forms of arthritis. Thus for the patient panel we focused on osteoarthritis, which is about ten times more prevalent than rheumatoid arthritis.

Provider Meeting

During the provider meeting, we had the opportunity to hear about several existing arthritis data bases. The Arthritis, Rheumatism, and Aging Medical Information System (ARAMIS) is based at Stanford University and has collected longitudinal data over 25 years in 11 sites across the United States and Canada. The data collection tools include standard clinical questions as well as a health assessment survey that includes items on disability, pain, and treatment side effects. Another existing data base, the National Databank for Rheumatic Diseases (NDB), is a research data base that collects information directly from patients with rheumatoid arthritis, osteoarthritis, and fibromyalgia. The NDB survey asks about pain, functional status, treatments, and comorbidities, among other things. These data bases would require substantial modification to produce outcomes data for osteoarthritis.

One clinical participant observed that many teaching hospitals are designing their own arthritis data bases for internal use. While these data bases are not designed for the purposes of shared decision-making, they might be modified in the future to support this purpose. Participants agreed that it would be difficult to ask patients to submit data to several different data bases; as a result, any effort to merge existing data collection efforts would be in everyone's best interest.

The provider group agreed that creating a new arthritis data base would be a difficult undertaking that would probably not be a very a useful tool for patients or their providers. This conclusion was driven by the belief that the data base would suffer from selection bias. Minimizing this bias would be challenging and require ongoing monitoring. Another challenge related to tracking outcomes from medication use among arthritis patients is that most people use several different courses of treatment from the time of diagnosis to the end of their life. New medications for the treatment of arthritis come on the market regularly and herbal remedies and other holistic approaches have become very popular. Therefore, patients' functional status and treatment decisions must be followed over many years in order to gather data that would be useful to others.

Another challenge is that the course of treatment is not linear. Not all patients progress from drug A to drug B to drug C to surgery, along with lifestyle modifications such as weight loss and exercise. Some patients may start with drug B or go straight to surgery or only use lifestyle changes as a method of treatment. Therefore, it might be difficult to assemble a sufficiently large cohort of people with the same demographic characteristics (e.g., age, race, and sex) who follow the same treatment course to predict differences in outcomes.

During the discussion regarding who should have access to such an outcomes data base, the provider group expressed quite a bit of doubt about the project. They felt that such a data base was unlikely to be very useful to patients, since it would be impossible to create a data base that was "all things to all people." Before starting, there should be some metric for defining success in order to evaluate the benefit of the project. The general consensus of the provider group seemed to be that piecing together some existing data bases might be useful, but starting from scratch was not.

Patient Focus Group

In contrast to the sentiments expressed by providers in the first consultative meeting, patients felt that an outcomes data base to help with treatment decisions would be extremely beneficial. Uniformly, the patient group wanted to know what people like them were experiencing and how other patients reacted to various treatments. Some of the patient participants felt that information was often difficult to find and that they did not know where to turn. Other patients stated that they had no difficulty finding the information they sought.

Some of the patients thought that a general data base that compiled information from a variety of sources would be useful—one that would lay out what the basic treatments are and when they are used. Such an information resource could contain information on different medications and their potential side effects, as well as lifestyle changes, holistic approaches, and surgical options. In addition, most patients felt that a "People Like Me" data base to compare outcomes from different treatments was exactly what was needed. This seemed to be especially true among patients who had already had joint replacement surgery or were considering it as an option. These patients indicated that it was difficult to assemble the information needed to make a treatment decision.

Though patients and providers differed in whether they thought a data base was a worthwhile effort, they did agree in some areas. Both groups felt that care would need to be taken in how the information was made available. Not all arthritis patients have access to the Internet, so while this may seem like a very easy way to get information to the largest number of people, other options such as brochures and disseminating information through providers would also need to be considered to enable patients to access the information. The same was noted for data collected from patients. A Web-based survey would likely be easier to implement than a paper-based one, but such an approach would miss a substantial number of potential respondents.

Patients and providers also agreed that any surveys to assess functioning and other outcomes would have to be short to minimize respondent burden and enhance the likelihood of participation; however, both groups agreed that patients would generally be willing to participate in such surveys. Patients in the group expressed a willingness to submit some information without compensation, although the more often a survey is required, the more likely that patients would ask for some compensation. If information comes mainly from patients, monetary compensation may not be necessary. It may be sufficient to offer newsletters or access to the data. If providers are required to input clinical information, they might expect monetary compensation to cover staff time for data entry.

While the groups expressed concern about the need for and feasibility of constructing a data base on arthritis treatments more generally, they supported a focus on evaluating patient outcomes for joint replacement surgery. The more-limited scope makes the concept more manageable and takes care of many of the concerns the provider group had regarding such a data base. Although patients may want more information than such a limited data base could provide, this seems to be an area where information is both lacking and needed.

There is a lack of information on comparative outcomes related to total joint replacement surgery for arthritis that patients can use to make informed decisions about whether to have joint replacement surgery and what they can expect from such treatment. For the remainder of this chapter, we focus our discussion on the feasibility issues associated with establishing a total joint replacement data base.

Issues Related to Establishing a Joint Replacement Data Base

Existing Data Base Efforts

In our review, we found only one United States-based data base on this topic. The Mayo Clinic has a data base that tracks patients who have undergone joint replacement surgery. Data are available on over 56,000 total joint replacements dating back to 1969, and the data base includes information on pain and functioning prior to the surgery as obtained by the physician and from the medical record. Operative notes provide information about the procedure, and reasons for surgery come from the medical record. Clinical results are collected through standardized surveys at one, two, and five years after the surgery and every five years after that. The entire system is computerized and automatically provides prompts for patient follow up at the appropriate intervals. The registry uses extensive methods to contact patients for follow up, including contacting them through social security numbers, relatives, nursing homes, or the post office. The data base does allow surgeons to query the information based on specific search parameters. This data base is the most promising prototype for a national arthritis outcomes data base. Currently, the Mayo Clinic data base does not allow patients access to the information, although staff at Mayo indicated they are interested in exploring the idea.

Outside the United States, several data bases track patients who have had joint replacement surgery, but the purpose of these data bases is not to track patient outcomes or to provide this information to patients and providers to assist with decisions about whether to have surgery or not.

Australia's National Joint Replacement Registry gathers information about patients while they are at the hospital for the surgery. The forms are completed while the patient is in the operating room and sent to the registry, usually in hard copy, though they are trying to move to electronic format. This registry's focus is on collecting the type of prostheses used in the surgery rather than the outcomes of surgery.

The province of Ontario, Canada, also has a joint registry. This data base does include some of the information of interest to a People Like Me outcomes data base, but the data base's primary purpose is to improve wait times and lower the rate of a second surgery. The Canadian data base variables include dates of referral, admission, and surgery; antibiotics ordered and administered; joint replaced; whether it is a primary or revision surgery; and the type of implant used. The physicians participating in the registry use hand-held computers to enter data in real time. The Ontario Ministry of Health and Long-term Care and the Ontario Orthopaedic Association cooperated to pilot the project in Southwestern Ontario.

The Swedish Knee Arthroplasty Registry (SKAR) has been tracking knee replacement surgeries and revisions since 1975. Primary knee replacement surgeries and revisions are reported annually to the Department of Orthopedics by the participating hospitals. The registry relies on the accuracy of the reported data from participating hospitals. The data base collects information regarding which knee is operated on, the date of operation, and information about the implant. There is no information on patient functional status, recovery time, or other data germane to tracking outcomes of treatment. In addition, about 20 percent of knee arthroplasties are not collected in the data base since the hospitals performing them do not participate in the project. A recent validation study found that about one-fifth of revisions from patients whose primary surgeries were included were not captured in the data base.

Approach to Collecting the Data

Outcomes data bases that rely primarily on patient input can be difficult to implement and maintain and are at risk of poor and incorrect recall of clinical details. Patients are a very good source of information on their experience with care and functioning pre- and posttreatment.

Many of the essential data elements for a joint replacement surgery outcomes data base can come directly from the physician, while others must come from the patient. Questions regarding a patient's height, weight, type of prosthesis, complications, and length of hospital stay are probably more accurate if they come from the physician. However, questions regarding pain, functional ability both before and after surgery, and demographic information would need to come from the patient. A key question for physicians involved in development would be to determine the time intervals for follow up with patients to assess the key outcomes of surgery—pain and level of functioning.

By collecting information only on those patients who undergo surgery, there is a slight advantage of being able to identify the patients and collect data from them at the outset of their treatment in relatively centralized locations (i.e., hospitals). Prior to surgery, patients could be given forms to complete to assess pretreatment pain and functioning. The hospital could also provide information on the surgical procedure and the device that is implanted. Once the patient leaves the hospital, this raises questions about the best mechanism(s) for collecting follow up information on pain and functioning posttreatment. Potential options include follow up directly with patients and follow up with the physicians who will provide them post-surgical care and observation.

Content of the Data Base

For the initial meeting with providers, we developed a draft set of questions of potential interest to patients and providers (see Appendix B). The questions were sent to participants prior to the meeting and discussed during the meeting. Since provider consensus from the first meeting was that another data base would not be useful for arthritis, the initial questions were put aside.

On further investigation, it was decided that a data base that tried to encompass all possible treatment options for arthritis would be extremely difficult and expensive to implement. For the patient focus group, the initial list of questions was pared down to only those relevant to patients with osteoarthritis. In contrast to physicians, patients did feel that an outcomes data base would be very helpful, especially for surgical treatment of arthritis.

Based on a narrowed list of questions focusing on joint replacement surgery for osteoarthritis, Table 5 contains a list of potential data elements for such a data base. Those marked with an asterisk could be gathered directly from the physician or hospital while those with double asterisks could probably be gathered through a standardized patient questionnaire at the hospital.

Table 5:

Illustrative Content of a Joint Replacement Surgery Outcomes Data Base

Category	Key Content
Patient Demographics	Date of birth* Gender* Race* Height/weight*
Pretreatment Pain and Functioning	Functional status prior to surgery** Changes in health habits prior to surgery** Pain prior to surgery** Devices/equipment used* Medication regimens**
Surgical Characteristics	Date of surgery* Specific joint replaced* Primary versus revision* Type of implant* Complications of surgery*
Acute and Postacute Hospital Care	Length of hospital stay Discharge location* Length of rehabilitation facility stay* Home health care received**
Posttreatment Recovery	Functional status assessments at routine intervals** Pain status assessments at routine intervals** Devices/equipment used* Medication regimens** Physical therapy*
Hospital Characteristics	Size* Ownership* Number of surgeries performed annually* Complication rates*
Surgeon Characteristics	Age* Specialty* Number of surgeries performed annually*

Instead of creating new questions to assess functional status, an option would be to use a standardized functional assessment questionnaire. The Western Ontario and McMaster Universities Arthritis Index (WOMAC) created by Nicholas Bellamy, et al. (1988) is considered the standard functional assessment for patients undergoing joint replacement surgery. The pain and functional status survey was originally developed in Canada and a version is now widely used in the United States as well. The questionnaire includes five questions about pain in the specified joint and 13 questions about difficulty with activities, both over the past week (see sample questions in Table 6). Each question is answered on a five-point scale, so that a simple sum gives a functional assessment score. Higher scores indicate more pain and more difficulty with

94

activities. The WOMAC could be administered before surgery and at specific intervals following surgery.

Table 6:
Sample WOMAC Questionnaire

 # 1. In the past week, how severe has your knee pain been?

(Circle one number on each line.)

	No pain	Mild pain	Moderate pain	Severe pain	Worst pain imagin-able	
a) At its worst?	1	2	3	4	5	V 1
b) Walking on a flat surface?	1	2	3	4	5	V 2
c) Going up or down stairs?	1	2	3	4	5	V 3
d) At night while in bed?	1	2	3	4	5	V 4
e) Sitting or lying	1	2	3	4	5	V 5

 # 2. In the past week, how much difficulty have you had with the following activities?

(Circle one number on each line.)

	No diffi-culty	Mild diffi-culty	Moderate difficulty	Severe diffi-culty	Could not do	
Going up stairs?	1	2	3	4	5	V 6
Going down stairs?	1	2	3	4	5	V 7
Walking on a flat surface?	1	2	3	4	5	V 8
Getting in and out of a car?	1	2	3	4	5	V 9
Going shopping?	1	2	3	4	5	V 10
Putting on shoes and socks?	1	2	3	4	5	V 11
Getting out of bed?	1	2	3	4	5	V 12
Getting in and out of bath?	1	2	3	4	5	V 13
Light housework or light yardwork?	1	2	3	4	5	V 14
Heavy housework or heavy yardwork?	1	2	3	4	5	V 15
Bicycling, hiking, or long walks?	1	2	3	4	5	V 16
Jogging or running?	1	2	3	4	5	V 17
Very strenuous sports?	1	2	3	4	5	V 18

Data Collection and Entry

The data base would likely evolve over time. The types of joint replacement surgeries and prostheses may change in the future. In addition, the format in which data are collected may change, especially if early iterations rely on paper questionnaires. For example, there might be a shift to an electronic format in the future.

Once data are entered into a specified format (Access Data base, Excel spreadsheet, etc.), raw data fields would need to be stored in such a way as to ensure flexibility in deriving final outcome fields and allowing analytic files to be constructed. In addition, data would need to be validated on a regular basis to verify that they are accurate.

Data collection must be simple and efficient in order to suit the needs of both those providing the data and those maintaining it. For providers, an electronic format, perhaps via the Internet, is probably most efficient. For patients, a solely electronic format may be more problematic since not everyone has access to the Internet. However, because all patients have to go through the hospital for their surgery, it may be feasible to supply the hospitals with a central terminal that patients can use to input data. This could be near the point of admission and discharge so that the questions are seamlessly integrated into these processes, perhaps as part of the presurgical work-up. An alternative is a paper survey that is administered during the presurgical work-up of the patient. For follow-up, a paper questionnaire would probably be best, although patients could be given a website where they could enter data electronically if they prefer.

Ensuring Participation

One of the challenges of creating the data base is recruiting of patients and physicians, both of whom will be asked to supply information. Establishing the osteoarthritis data base will require the inclusion of all of the providers who see the patient, from the time of the treatment decision through the surgery. Given the need to establish the baseline functioning of the patient prior to surgery, it would be necessary to recruit patients through their doctors and enroll patients at the time the decision is made to have surgery. Additionally, it would be necessary to recruit the participation of hospitals and surgeons, who will need to provide information to the data base. Patients are more likely to agree to participate if their providers agree to participate and are willing to endorse the project. Hospitals are likely to be willing to provide their own data if they get something in return. Some may insist on payment for the time needed to enter the data in whatever form requested. Others may be willing to provide data in exchange for access to the aggregate data. They may find a benefit to being able to compare their outcomes to those on a regional or national level.

Recruiting patients in the hospital may be the best method for ensuring their participation. This may provide the easiest access to patients, and collecting data at discharge would allow for collection of the maximum amount of information at one time. However, this approach may not be sufficient for capturing all the information required prior to surgery. Because follow-up surveys are required, patient buy-in to the data base concept must be established to encourage ongoing participation. Patient participants in our focus group indicated that they would be willing to provide information for such a data base because it would help others experiencing the same problems in the future and because they would want to have access to the data if they ever needed it in the future.

Sponsorship and Funding

A data base such as the one proposed is a difficult and expensive undertaking. Without sponsorship of a reputable organization and adequate funding, the data base will never become operational. Start-up costs for such a project can be significant, so substantial funding must be provided at the outset for the planning and pilot phases as well as the initiation of the large-scale data base.

Patients in our focus group mentioned the Arthritis Foundation (AF) as a sponsoring organization that they would trust. Since the AF is the only national patient advocacy group dedicated to problems associated with osteoarthritis, it is a logical host for the information and one of a potential consortium of sponsors. The AF is dedicated to ensuring that patients are able to obtain the necessary information to deal with their disease, so an outcomes data base on joint replacement surgery is consistent with the organization's aims.

The National Institute of Arthritis and Musculoskeletal and Skin Diseases (NIAMS) at the National Institutes of Health (NIH) is a potential funder. However, we heard from some patients that they would prefer to have a nongovernmental organization behind the information they receive. Therefore, while NIAMS is a very good source of funding, a combination of the two organizations might be best to ensure that patients trust the source enough to provide data.

Constructing the Information Tool

Once the data are compiled for the purposes of determining whether patients experience differences in outcomes from surgical treatment, the next challenge is packaging the information in a way that is usable for consumers and physicians. The approach to organizing and displaying the information needs to be given considerable thought and testing, as the cognitive psychology and decision-making sciences literature finds that the way information is framed and the complexity of the data display affect whether the information is used to make decisions and what choices are made (Slovic, 1995; Hibbard et al., 2002). How the material is presented (e.g., mortality versus survival) can influence individual decisions about which treatment to choose; consequently, it is important that the direction and the extent of the influence of the display formats be known and defensible. A key responsibility of the information producer is to produce information that can be used by consumers for choice but will not influence their decision-making in unintended ways. This will require mocking up various prototypes of the decision tool and testing them with patients for design influences—in addition to standard cognitive testing for comprehension and usability. Developers of the consumer information platform will also need to be sensitive to the presentation of complex information for audiences with varying levels of literacy.

As use of the Internet increases and given the structure of Web-based platforms for disseminating information—which allow for easier and cheaper approaches to tailoring information to individual users—the decision aid tool derived from a People Like Me national data base would likely be a computer-based platform. A computer-assisted decision tool can potentially help with the challenge consumers face in processing and weighing various factors to make a choice—especially if the information is tailored to their own situation. While a computer platform may work for a majority of users, the developers will need to better understand what avenues and preferences consumers have for accessing the information (e.g., print materials, video tapes), because not all patients and their families will have access to the Internet.

The time it takes to develop a computer-aided decision tool will need to be factored into the overall project timeline; this product by itself will likely take two to three years to develop.

Feasibility Issues

Bias

It would be nearly impossible and very expensive to recruit, gain consent, and track all 435,000 Americans who have joint replacement surgery each year. As a result, the data base would need to focus on a sample of the population of patients who undergo surgery, with the goal of working to ensure that the sample of patients who participate in the data base is representative of the population of patients undergoing joint replacement surgery. Given the voluntary nature of participation in an outcomes data base, it would be important to obtain basic demographic and clinical information on patients who do not want to be tracked to test for bias and to understand which patients are underrepresented. It may be necessary to implement strategies to actively recruit subgroups that are underrepresented in the data base.

Sample Size

The actual sample size needed to allow adequate power for reasonable comparisons varies depending on how many comparisons we wish to make. For each category, to detect a difference of 20 percentage points without any further interaction would only require a sample size of 99 per category. On the other hand, to detect a difference of 5 percentage points with interactions between variables, we would need a sample size of 3,139 per category. Assuming that the variables are perfectly balanced (i.e., half of the values are high, half of the values are low) and the worst-case scenario of probabilities of interest at 0.5, then a sample size of 3,925 patients would be required under the following situation: a 10-percentage-point difference in outcomes of interest, the presence of two-level interaction terms, and the variable with the largest number of categories is five (e.g., race/ethnicity) —so 5 x 785 (per Table 3). For a case with only a 5-percentage-point difference in outcomes and interaction effects, we now need 3,139 patients per cell, so 5 x 3,139 = 15,695.

Endpoints

There are several endpoints that patients are interested in including surgical complications, functional ability after the surgery, and level of pain. The starting point is the baseline functional status and level of pain prior to surgery at the point the treatment decision is made. Postsurgery outcomes are both those that occur in the near term and the long-term. Joint replacement prostheses usually last about 10 years and then the patient often needs a second surgery—which suggests the need for a follow-up period of at least 10 years. However, researchers who have tracked patients longitudinally report difficulties staying in contact with patients and gaining their cooperation in responding to inquiries for information over long periods of time. As a result, careful thought needs to be given to determine the best strategies for following patients to capture long-term outcomes. In terms of immediate changes in functioning, the most pertinent information can be gleaned within a couple years of the surgery—so follow ups at six-month intervals for the first two years postsurgery are probably sufficient.

Outputs

Reports could be generated from these data by subgroups: age, sex, and functional status. We do not suggest attempting to cut the data more finely since small numbers in each cell will likely lead to uninterpretable information. However, within these groups, we would suggest making the reports as tailored as possible to accommodate various end users, although this may be more expensive to maintain.

Clinical and Patient Input into Design

To begin with, a set of clinical experts should be convened to agree on the content of the data base and the measurement strategy. In particular, clinical input will be important with the functional status measurement and the outcomes that the data base will track. However, clinician input is not sufficient. We will also need input from patients who may use the data base. If doctors are only interested in tracking complications from surgery but patients are really interested in functional status after surgery, that will need to be addressed. On the other hand, if patients ignore the possibility of complications, that does not mean that the data base should ignore them since they are a factor in recovery. The data base must serve the needs of all key stakeholders (i.e., those who supply and use the information). Thus, the union of data elements required by potential participants will be necessary.

Clinicians are essential for defining the technical aspects of the data base and getting buy-in from the physicians likely to provide data. They are also the best source for identifying the time periods of interest. Psychometric experts should be consulted to determine the costs and benefits associated with different follow-up periods.

Confidentiality

Anytime someone gives personal information to someone else, confidentiality is an issue. In this case, we would need to collect contact information, including name, address, and possibly telephone number, to administer follow-up surveys. Therefore, each patient should be assigned a research ID number when he or she completes the initial questionnaire. This way, information regarding functional status and outcomes can be kept separate from contact information, ensuring that people accessing the data base cannot obtain contributors' contact information. Patients must be assured that all data will remain confidential and that others will only be able to access data in aggregate form. This is standard for most research projects, so confidentiality should not present a larger problem than it would in other projects. In fact, we are not suggesting collecting much information that could be considered sensitive, so it is unlikely that patients would be unduly concerned about confidentiality.

On the other hand, if data were collected through the Centers for Medicare and Medicaid Services (CMS), it is probable that we would need to keep social security numbers on file as well. This makes confidentiality more problematic. If the project were somehow government sponsored, respondents may be willing to be tracked by social security number, but people are generally very wary about giving out this information. If data can be collected and matched with other data elements without collecting social security numbers, we would advise this.

Timeline

There are quite a few steps involved in creating a new outcomes data base. Table 7 below summarizes the key steps and estimates of the time required to build a data base.

Table 7:

Timeline and Key Milestones for Developing Data Base Prototype

Key Milestones	Timeline
I. Planning Stage	
Define purpose of data base, who will use information, and how that information will be disseminated.	Months 1 - 3
Identify key constituencies that need to be collaborators in the project (e.g., Arthritis Foundation, American College of Rheumatology, National Institute of Arthritis and Musculoskeletal and Skin Diseases, Centers for Medicare and Medicaid Services). Solicit feedback, input, and support from appropriate patient and provider constituency groups as well as hospitals; begin to lay groundwork for working collaboratively with these groups to promote the benefits of participating in the data base and securing the commitment of physicians and patients to supply data, especially through hospital contacts or through CMS.	Months 1 - 12
Refine the set of questions the data base will seek to answer and engage patients, clinicians, and researchers in a consensus development exercise to specify and define the set of outcome measures that will be measured and reported to patients and physicians.	Months 1 - 12
Define and gain consensus from the patient, clinical, and research communities on the set of stratifying variables (covariates) that are predictive factors in determining outcomes and that patients will be able to use to query the data base to get answers for "People Like Me." Patients who are undergoing joint replacement surgery should be asked to specify how they would like to query the data.	Months 1 - 12
Review existing data collection efforts and the published literature to determine which questions can be answered already by the relevant "People Like Me" subsetting variables. Grade the level of evidence contained in the research studies. Identify where the gaps remain that a new data base effort could fill. Seek to construct a collaborative pooling of data across data collection efforts so as to be able to conduct cross-site analyses, and to standardize data definitions, data collection tools, and outcomes of interest.	Months 1 - 18
Define the mechanisms for collecting the data (survey, administrative data, chart abstraction).	Months 12 - 24
Define the sampling method for selecting physicians and patients, possibly by hospital.	Months 12 - 18
Take the "key questions" to be addressed by the data base and define the set of data elements required and operationalize the definitions. Identify the data source and frequency of collection for each element. Determine whether new data collection tools are required or whether existing tools can be modified.	Months 12 - 24
Prepare training materials (training manual, data code book).	Months 20 - 24
Beta-test data entry procedures and data definitions.	Months 20 - 24

Table 7 – Continued

Key Milestones	Timeline
Design a pilot test of the data collection tools and processing protocols.	Months 18 - 24
II. Pilot Stage	
Identify a small number of practice sites (<=5) to pilot test the data collection methodology.	Month 24
Train pilot site personnel on data collection methods.	Months 24 - 25
Commence data collection in pilot sites.	Months 25 - 36
Interview staff at each of the practice sites to identify what worked and did not work during pilot implementation.	Months 30 - 36
Review data that are submitted to assess completeness, consistency, and accuracy.	Months 26 - 36
Revise data collection tools and procedures.	Months 36 - 37
III. Full-Scale Implementation of Data Collection	
Expand data collection to more practice sites—recruit providers and patients into the study.	Months 38 - 54
Conduct training of personnel in each site on the data collection.	Months 38 - 54
Begin collecting data; provide technical assistance to sites.	Months 39 +
IV. Data Analysis	
Data processing protocols—data cleaning, auditing, analysis.	Months 39 +
Organize results for distribution to providers and patients.	Months 48 +
V. Development of Information/Decision Support Tool	
Meet with patient representatives to define the content of the information resource and how it should be communicated.	Months 12 - 15
Meet with physician representatives to define the information they would like to see presented for use by physicians to assist with making treatment decisions.	Months 15 - 18
Review the cognitive literature on consumer/patient decision-making to guide the design of the information resource.	Months 15 - 20
Develop a mock-up of a prototype decision support tool for review by patients and physicians.	Months 20 - 26
Conduct testing with patients/consumers for design influences (e.g., framing, use of language), comprehension, and usability.	Months 26 - 30
Build consumer information tool.	Months 36 - 48
VI. Dissemination/Public Awareness	
Build awareness among the patient and provider community that a tool is available to assist with making treatment decisions (public education campaign).	Months 48 - 56

Costs

The cost of developing a data base in the United States is difficult to determine. The Australia project collects data from 296 hospitals, or 100 percent of hospitals performing joint replacement surgery. Australia performed a pilot project in the southern part of the country in 1998 and began collecting data from all hospitals in 2001. The Australian government funds the registry, and it has a budget of approximately $1.5 million to cover the period from 1998 to 2005. This covers salary for one coordinator, a computer programmer, a data manager, a part-time statistician, and 6 - 7 full-time-equivalent data entry people. A committee of volunteers oversees the project, and there is one coordinator at each hospital who does not receive any compensation.

It is unlikely that this budget would be large enough for a project of this magnitude here, however. Approximately 40,000 joint replacement surgeries are performed in Australia a year, compared to 435,000 in the United States. On a per-person basis, this would mean a tenfold increase in costs for a comparable effort in the United States. As noted earlier, an alternative approach would be to sample from the total number of joint replacement surgeries. Assuming inclusion of 100 percent of all cases in the United States, an upper bound estimate might approach $10.5 million. Additionally, start-up costs of establishing the data base are likely to be quite high, but the incremental cost of each additional person's data beyond some minimum is not likely to be that large.

The Swedish registry estimates that its data collection costs about $40 per patient per entry (either for primary or revision surgery), but it does not follow up unless there is a revision. These costs are likely to be much lower than costs for a data base here. The Mayo Clinic estimates that its data base has an administrative cost of about $400,000 per year. However, even though their methods are closer to what we are proposing, given that they have a ready-made base for data collection, this, too, is likely to be low.

Patient Information Page

The following is the information page that the Australian Orthopaedic Association National Joint Replacement Registry gives to patients when they are attempting to procure patient consent. Offering information like this could be helpful in getting patients to participate in and consent to providing their data to an arthritis surgery outcomes data base. The information sheet would need to make clear what data were being requested from the patient and for what purposes, as this "patient information" sheet does. In the case of establishing an arthritis surgery outcomes data base, the notice should make it clear that patient's name and address are being collected solely for the purposes of conducting important follow up surveys to track long-term outcomes (i.e., functional status) and will not be stored with survey data for others to view.

Our focus would clearly be different because our proposed data base would look at outcomes rather than just register the type of prosthesis used. An information sheet could also be an opportunity to appeal to patients to help others undergoing joint replacement in the future by providing data that others could use to make decisions and gather information about the surgery. Finally, it is a way to explain how data will be collected and the procedure that will be used to ensure that it will be kept confidential, in the hope of further encouraging participation.

INTRODUCTION—about the Registry

You are about to have a hip or knee replacement. This operation is very successful and most people do not require any further surgery following this procedure. However, a number of people who have a joint replacement may at some time in the future require another operation on that joint. This may occur due to a variety of reasons; the most common being that the joint replacement has worn out. Furthermore, differences between the many types of artificial joints available may affect the time at which they wear out and require replacing. In order to improve the success of this surgery, the Australian Orthopaedic Association has set up a National Joint Replacement Registry so that joint replacement and prostheses can be monitored. The purpose of the registry is to record information on every person having a joint replacement. Approximately 40,000 people have joint replacement surgery each year in Australia. It is also important to record details on any subsequent operations and the reason the surgery was performed. By analyzing this information it will be possible to identify the cause of any problems as well as determine which types of joint replacement have the best results. To be successful, the registry needs to gather information on as many people having hip or knee replacement surgery as possible. We are asking you to participate in the registry, by allowing us to document information relevant to your operation.

Your Involvement—the information we need

The information we require includes your name, date of birth, address, Medicare number, hospital identity number, the name of the hospital, and the reason you are having a joint replacement. This information is necessary to accurately link you to the artificial joint inserted, as well as linking any following joint surgery you may have to your previous records. We will also record the day of the operation, which joint was operated on, and the type of artificial joint used. No other personal information is recorded. Hospitals and government will send reports to the registry on a regular basis to validate the information collected.

Information—how we will keep your information confidential

Your personal information is confidential and cannot be used outside the registry. Procedures are in place to protect your information and to keep it confidential. When your details have been entered into the registry your record will be given a specific registry number. In addition you cannot be identified in any reports produced by the registry.

How we will collect the information

Although we are asking to record your operation details in the registry you are not required to do anything. Your surgeon and/or theatre staff will complete the form that contains your personal details at the time of your operation and send it to us. The information will be entered into the registry computer.

Risks and Benefits—to you

There are no risks to you by having your details in the registry. Your information is protected and we are not allowed to identify you by law. The registry will produce general reports on a variety of factors that influence the success of joint replacement surgery. This will improve the quality of future joint replacement surgery.

How to remove your name from the registry

We understand that not everyone is comfortable about having his or her personal details documented in a registry. If you feel this way and do not want your details recorded please contact the Project Coordinator. A decision on whether or not you wish to be involved in the registry does not affect your treatment in any way.

Source: Australian Orthopaedic Association National Joint Replacement and Registry

CHAPTER 6:
CONCLUSIONS AND RECOMMENDATIONS

Is There a Need for National Outcomes Data Bases?

Based on our review of prostate cancer and osteoarthritis as two candidate clinical conditions that illustrate the complexity of treatment choices faced by patients, we found a very strong desire among patients to have access to an information source that would not only explain what their condition is but would also help them understand what the various treatment options are and what outcomes (i.e., survival, functioning, side effects) people like themselves could expect from each of the various treatment options. Overwhelmingly, patients observed that information on differences between treatment options and outcomes was difficult to obtain, was not synthesized and presented in a way to allow them to understand the tradeoffs, and rarely offered insights as to what their own experience might be given their unique patient characteristics (e.g., age, race/ethnicity, gender, health status, stage of disease). Patients also underscored that they do not have a reliable source for accurate information on alternative treatment therapies and their effectiveness, something that is of high interest to patients. Patients with prostate cancer and osteoarthritis also described relying heavily on other patients for information—in the absence of information that was presented from the patient's perspective as to what they might experience—as well as the Internet, where they acknowledged it was difficult to assess the accuracy of the information presented.

Patients, perhaps because of their own difficulties in finding information, indicated they would be very willing to participate in a longitudinal outcomes data base, particularly if they understood that it would benefit future patients in their quest for information. While patients wanted to ensure that their own personal data were protected, they did not see privacy issues as an obstacle to their participation. Patients expressed a preference for the federal government (e.g., National Institutes of Health) or a nationally respected and trusted organization (e.g., American Cancer Society) to operate such a system because these parties would have no vested interest in any particular form of treatment and were more likely to present accurate information. Patients noted they would have reservations about participating if the project were sponsored and operated by a pharmaceutical company or medical device manufacturer that produces a treatment. Their concern stemmed from a belief that these types of entities might be less willing to provide objective information and/or might try to market products directly to patients participating in the data base project.

Providers also expressed considerable support for the People Like Me data base concept, particularly as it pertained to obtaining information on the clinical benefits of various therapies for different types of patients. They also seemed interested in finding ways to better organize and present information to help patients understand treatment options because they currently struggle with how best to communicate with patients given a wide range of abilities and patient preferences for information—from "you make the decision, doctor" to "I want to know all my choices and what is going to happen as a result of each choice." Both providers and patients agreed that a national outcomes data base would provide an important tool for shared decision-making between patients and providers, something that is currently lacking.

Providers did express concern about the validity of the data base depending on how the sample of patients whose data make up the data base were chosen. They underscored the complexity of gaining representative participation by providers and patients in a voluntary data base that reflected a sample of patients with the condition—which could potentially lead to a biased sample. Physicians expressed some reservations about patients being able to view the outcomes information by themselves outside of the doctor-patient consultation; however, they acknowledged that the Internet has greatly transformed the discussions that doctors have with their patients—so that patients often come to the doctor armed with information they want to discuss. Their primary concern regarding the construction of the data base seemed to be with the accuracy and validity of the information contained in the system.

Is It Feasible to Develop a National Outcomes Data Base?

With respect to the feasibility of developing national outcomes data bases, it was clear from our research that efforts have already been made—both in the United States and abroad—to develop data collection systems that longitudinally track patient outcomes. Outside the United States, these are more frequently disease registries that capture 100 percent of the patients with a particular condition or treatment—typically within national health systems. The information derived from the longitudinal data base systems that we reviewed was viewed as extremely valuable for research purposes to understand how patients fare under different forms of treatment—especially as treatments evolve after the clinical trial stage. And, while not yet fully realizing their potential in this regard, the data bases were seen as a valuable tool to support clinicians in their interactions with patients. None of the projects that we reviewed had taken the next step of making the information available for direct use by patients, although the developers noted that this was an important audience for the information, and they were interested in finding ways to translate existing data for use by consumers and exploring how they might modify their data base efforts in the future to support greater shared decision-making between physicians and patients.

The existing longitudinal data base efforts demonstrate that establishing an outcomes data base is technically feasible and is valued by end users, but that substantial resources are required to design and operate them. The amount of resources required largely depends on the number of patients and providers required to participate in the data base to produce statistically reliable results by different profiles of interest to patients (how many People Like Me demographic and clinical characteristics are accounted for), the amount of data required to be captured (how many data elements), the frequency and intensity of follow up efforts to track patients over time, and the scope of the effort (how many conditions and interventions are being monitored). To establish and operate a national outcomes data base, the investment is likely to range from $5 to $25 million annually—with the costs determined by the factors noted above.

Summary

Based on discussions with patients and clinicians, it is clear that comparative outcome information is lacking for many treatments and that patients make difficult decisions every day with little or poor information to inform those choices. We also know from the studies on shared decision-making tools that the availability of and promotion of the use of such tools can encourage greater information-sharing between patients and providers and help patients make more informed decisions and feel more satisfied with decisions. We also acknowledge that not all medical conditions would be appropriate for developing a longitudinal outcomes data base that could be used by patients and their physicians. As noted in Chapter 2, we outline key criteria that should be evaluated in the process of selecting appropriate conditions for such an effort. It is also important to note that the construction of such a data base will be complex and will benefit from starting with a pilot to test the concept and the design of the systems used to capture the data and then expanding over time to build the information base. Also, it appears that given the broad array of individuals—physicians, medical organizations, patients, and researchers—who will need to be involved, the effort will be most likely to succeed if it is a consortium effort.

There is keen interest among patients to have a People Like Me resource, providers support this activity, and smaller-scale efforts have been successfully designed and implemented. Prior to undertaking the establishment of any national outcomes data base, we recommend conducting meetings with patient and provider representatives to solicit their support for and input into the design of the system. While various health conditions share similar features, we did identify through the patient-provider discussions some unique factors across different conditions that would affect the design and implementation of an outcomes data base. The patient and provider meetings and ongoing involvement will be essential steps in firmly defining the scope of the project, the goals of the data base, how data will be captured (which outcomes are of interest and how are they measured), how the data are analyzed, and how and what data will be shared with patients and providers—and will increase the chances of successful development and implementation.

Patient Questions

Treatment

1. When is surgery a preferable intervention for prostate cancer ("PC"), and when is radiation treatment preferable? Are there *any* clear tradeoffs between these two treatment options?

2. Does my age, ethnicity, medical history, or PC status (i.e., Gleason score, clinical stage, PSA level) modify the likely outcomes for the different forms of treatment?

3. When is "watchful waiting" a reasonable treatment option?

4. What is the likelihood of a "cure," for each kind of treatment?

5. What is the difference between "external beam radiation therapy" and "brachytherapy" (implant therapy)? Is there a survival advantage for preferring one to the other, either in general or based on age, ethnicity, PC status (i.e., Gleason score, clinical stage, PSA level), etc.? What are the side effects associated with brachytherapy?

6. What are the differences between the various forms of external beam radiation therapy for PC, such as 3-D conformal therapy, IMRT, and proton beam therapy? Do any of these offer a survival advantage?

7. Is cryotherapy a reasonable treatment alternative for PC? What are the side effects and survival data regarding cryotherapy?

8. What about hormone treatment for PC? When is hormone treatment appropriate as an adjunct to radiation, and how much does it improve survival?

9. What about experimental treatments, like genetic therapy or Endostatin (anti-angiogenic drugs)? Are these treatments available, safe, and effective (by comparison with surgery and radiation)?

10. What about "alternative treatments" for PC (e.g., herbal remedies, PC-SPES, etc.)? Are these treatments safe, and are they effective (either by themselves, or as a supplement to medical or surgical treatment)?

11. What is the likelihood of tumor recurrence following PC treatment that initially appears to be successful? Does this vary based on treatment type, age, ethnicity, PC status (i.e., Gleason score, clinical stage, PSA level, etc.)?

12. How can I get quantitative information to compare survival rates across different forms of treatment, for men with different ages, ethnicities, medical histories, PC status (i.e., Gleason score, clinical stage, PSA level, etc.)? Does my doctor have access to such information?

Side Effects

1. What is the likelihood of impotence as a side effect? Does this likelihood vary by type of treatment or by patient characteristics?

2. What is the likelihood of urinary incontinence as a side effect? Does this likelihood vary by type of treatment or by type of patient?

3. What is the likelihood of bowel dysfuction (e.g., diarrhea, constipation, fecal incontinence) as a side effect? Does this likelihood vary by type of treatment or by patient characteristics?

4. What other side effects should I anticipate as a function of treatment? Do these vary either by treatment type or by patient characteristics?

5. With regard to any side effects of treatment, what is the likely duration, level of impairment, and prognosis for improvement? Are there secondary therapies available to ameliorate side effects (e.g., Viagra)?

Assessment

1. What is a Gleason Grade, and what does my Gleason score tell me about my PC?

2. What is the "Prostate Specific Antigen" (PSA) test? What does my PSA score tell me about my PC?

3. What is a "Digital Rectal Examination" (DRE)? What does DRE tell me about my PC?

4. What other sorts of diagnostic testing are commonly used for PC patients? Are there specific diagnostic tests that I should ask my doctor to perform?

5. What are the Partin Nomograms? How do I use the Partin Nomograms, and how can they help me to make decisions about treatment?

6. How do I use my assessment information in making decisions about treatment? Is there a relationship between my assessment scores and positive outcomes (or survival rates) for the different sorts of therapy?

Sources of Care

1. Are some doctors or medical facilities better than others at administering surgical or radiation treatment for PC? How do I pick the right care provider for me?

2. Should I plan on obtaining multiple medical opinions before pursuing treatment? What are the differences between oncologists and urologists, and whom should I see first?

3. What should I do if my health plan doesn't cover the treatment option that I feel is best for me?

Behavioral Interventions

1. Does diet protect against the development of PC, and can dietary factors help to promote recovery from PC? If so, what dietary factors are important? Is there evidence to show improved survival as a function of diet?

2. Does exercise protect against the development of PC, or promote recovery from PC? Is there evidence to show improved survival as a function of exercise?

3. Are there any other things that I can do, apart from diet and exercise, in order to promote wellness and recovery from PC? Is there evidence to show improved PC survival based on any behavioral or interpersonal factors, apart from diet and exercise?

Social Support

1. What are the emotional side effects of PC treatment? Do these vary by type of treatment, type of patient, etc.?

2. What sorts of support resources are available to me? Should I consider joining a PC support group?

3. What support resources are available for my spouse and family?

Provider Questions

Communication Issues

1. What kind of survival information do PC patients need? Where do I obtain such information, and how do I convey it most effectively to my patients?

2. How do I talk with patients about the likelihood of a "cure" for their PC? How can I communicate information about recurrence, survival rates, and mortality in a manner that is at once objectively accurate, sympathetic, and reassuring?

3. How much information and counseling should I provide to patients in making their PC treatment decisions? To what extent are tradeoffs between survival and side effects a matter of individual preference, as opposed to objectively available information? What can I do to make my patients' decisions easier?

Treatment

1. Is there evidence to support any clear decision rule for choosing between surgery and radiation treatment for PC, for any set of patients with the disease, based on demographics, PC status (i.e., Gleason score, clinical stage, PSA level), medical history, etc.? If so, what is the rule?

2. What are the survival rates for surgical and radiation treatments for PC, with conditional probabilities based on demographics, PC status (i.e., Gleason score, clinical stage, PSA level), medical history, etc.?

3. When is "watchful waiting" a reasonable treatment option? What are the survival rates for watchful waiting, with conditional probabilities based on demographics, PC status (i.e., Gleason score, clinical stage, PSA level), medical history, etc.?

4. Is there any survival basis for preferring external beam radiation therapy to brachytherapy, either in general or based on age, ethnicity, PC status (i.e., Gleason score, clinical stage, PSA level), etc.?

5. When is hormone treatment for PC an appropriate adjunct to radiation, by how much does it improve survival rates, and for what sorts of patients?

6. What about experimental treatments, like genetic therapy or Endostatin (anti-angiogenic drugs)? Are these treatments available, safe, and effective (by comparison with surgery and radiation)? Is there any survival data available on new, experimental forms of treatment?

7. What about "alternative treatments" for PC (e.g., herbal remedies, PC-SPES)? Are these treatments safe, and are they effective (either by themselves, or as a supplement to medical or surgical treatment)? Is there any survival data available on alternative treatments?

8. What is the likelihood of tumor recurrence following PC treatment that initially appears to be successful? Does recurrence vary based on treatment type, age, ethnicity, PC status (i.e., Gleason score, clinical stage, PSA level), etc.?

Side Effects

1. What is the likelihood of impotence as a side effect, with conditional probabilities based on type of treatment and patient characteristics?

2. What is the likelihood of urinary incontinence as a side effect, with conditional probabilities based on type of treatment and patient characteristics?

3. What is the likelihood of bowel dysfunction as a side effect, with conditional probabilities based on type of treatment and patient characteristics?

4. What other side effects should PC patients anticipate as a function of particular forms of treatment, and how common are such side effects? Do these vary either by treatment type or by patient characteristics?

5. With regard to all side effects associated with each form of treatment, what is the likely duration, level of impairment, and prognosis for improvement? Are there secondary therapies available to ameliorate treatment side effects (e.g., Viagra)?

Draft Questions—Arthritis Consultative Meeting;
March 13, 2002

Patient Questions

General Treatment Questions

1. Will these treatments (drugs/physical therapy/other) stop or slow the progress of my arthritis?

2. What should I expect from these treatments? For example, how effective are they in helping my pain and stiffness? Do they work immediately? For how long are they likely to be effective? Can I stop treatment when I start to feel better?

3. Will I be able to function normally while I am on these drugs? Will I be able to do all of the tasks of daily living? Will I be able to exercise?

4. Does the kind of treatment I choose depend on whether I have other health problems?

Drug Therapy

1. Which drugs would be best for me to take? How soon will I feel better? Will I be able to resume my normal activities? How does my type of arthritis affect the treatment options that are available to me?

2. Can I take just one of these drugs or will I have to take more than one?

3. How difficult is to follow the instructions for each of the drugs I might take? For example, how often do the pills have to be taken? Do some have to be taken with or without food? Do some require that I have blood taken to check for any problems? Will I have to have other tests done (bone density test for example)?

4. Are there over-the-counter medications I should avoid when I am taking these arthritis medications?

Other Treatments

1. When should I consider surgery? Are there different types of surgeries available? How well do they work? Will I be cured? What are the risks of these surgeries?

Side Effects

1. What types of side effects am I likely to have from taking any of the arthritis drugs?

2. How likely is it that I will have stomach or intestinal side effects such as ulcers or serious bleeding with different treatments? Are some people at greater risk of having problems?

3. How likely is it that I will have problems with my kidneys or liver if I take each of these treatments? Are some people at greater risk of having problems?

4. Is there a risk of death associated with any of these side effects? If so, how high is this risk? Are some people more likely to die?

5. Can the seriousness or occurrence of these side effects be limited or prevented? Will they stop if I stop taking the treatment?

6. Are there things I will not be able to do (eat certain foods, drink alcohol, engage in physical activities)?

Self-Care Strategies

1. How effective are diet and exercise in treating my arthritis?

2. Is there anything I can do to minimize flare-ups?

3. Will taking vitamins or other supplements help me?

4. Are different exercises recommended for different types of arthritis?

5. Are there activities I should avoid?

6. What changes in my life or environment should I make to slow down the disease and maintain my ability to do my normal activities?

7. Are there devices or products that can help me feel better or perform daily tasks more easily?

Psychosocial Support

1. What types of community resources are available to me?

2. Do support groups help? Are some better than others?

Provider Questions

Communication

1. How can I tell my patients enough about the disease and its treatments to know what to expect and to make decisions without overwhelming them or causing unnecessary anxiety?

2. How do I communicate the uncertainty associated with treatment effectiveness and disease progression?

3. What questions should I be asking my patients to make sure that I give them the information that is most relevant for them?

4. How much do the information needs about treatment options, self-care management strategies, and community resources vary by patient characteristics such as age, gender, arthritis severity, functional ability, family income and available social support?

5. How can I make sure that my patients fully understand the information they have received?

6. How can I accurately assess my patients' level of pain and function?

Treatment

1. What is the evidence base for the different types of arthritis treatments including drugs, surgery, physical/occupational therapy, and education? Is this evidence base equally applicable to all types of patients?

2. Are different drugs within a major class (e.g., NSAIDs) equally effective? Is there evidence to suggest differential effectiveness in different types of patients?

3. What are the risks and benefits associated with surgery? Do these risks and benefits vary by patient characteristics such as age, gender, type of arthritis, etc.?

4. What recommendations should I make regarding alternative or complementary therapies? Is there an evidence base for any of these recommendations? Are the risk/benefit tradeoffs for these treatments comparable for all patients?

Side Effects

1. Do different drugs within a major class (e.g., NSAIDs) produce similar side effects? Are the risks of side effects similar for drugs in the same class? Are the risks similar for patients with different characteristics?

2. What are the rates of occurrence for gastrointestinal and other side effects with the different types of treatment? Are they similar for patients with different characteristics?

Self-Care Strategies

1. Is there evidence that self care strategies work for this disease? How do I encourage compliance with self-care strategies, such as a regular exercise regimen and a weight reduction plan?

2. Is there a trusted resource I can recommend to my patients to find devices and products that can help them perform routine tasks? Where can I find information regarding their effectiveness?

Specific Additional Questions for Rheumatoid Arthritis

Patient Questions

1. Will these treatments (drugs/physical therapy/other) stop or slow the progress of my arthritis?

2. What should I expect from these treatments? For example, how effective are they in helping my pain and stiffness? Do they work immediately? For how long are they likely to be effective? Can I stop treatment when I start to feel better?

3. Will I be able to function normally while I am on these drugs? Will I be able to do all of the tasks of daily living? Will I be able to exercise?

4. How difficult is it to follow the instructions for each of the drugs I might take? For example, how often do the pills have to be taken? Do some have to be taken with or without food? Do some require that I have blood taken to check for any problems? Will I have to have other tests done (bone density test for example)?

5. Are there any special medical considerations that I need to take into account because of my RA (i.e., patients with RA should get a pneumovax and flu shot every year, but patients on immunosuppresives should not get live vaccines)?

Provider Questions

1. How do I best assess disease activity and response to therapy?

2. What is the evidence base for the different types of arthritis treatments including drugs, surgery, physical/occupational therapy, and education? Is this evidence base equally applicable to all types of patients?

3. Are different drugs within a major class (e.g., NSAIDs) equally effective? Is there evidence to suggest differential effectiveness in different types of patients?

4. What recommendations should I make regarding alternative or complementary therapies? Is there an evidence base for any of these recommendations? Are the risk/benefit tradeoffs for these treatments comparable for all patients?

Surgery Questions

1. What is total joint replacement?
   Why is total joint replacement necessary?

2. Are there any alternatives to having surgery?
   What joints can be replaced?

3. What is the implant itself like?

4. What is it made of?

5. Will I be able to tell it is artificial once I recover from surgery?

6. How is total joint replacement done?

7. What will happen during my recovery from total joint replacement?

8. What do I need to do to prepare for recovery?

9. How long will recovery take?

10. How painful will recovery be?

11. How difficult will it be to walk or do other activities once I have joint replacement surgery?

12. What are the possible complications from total joint replacement?

13. How common is: Infection? Blood clotting? Loosening of the joint? Dislocation of the joint? Wear on the joint? Prosthetic breakage? Nerve injury?

14. Is total joint replacement permanent?

15. Will the joint ever have to be replaced again?

16. What medical information do I need to collect before my surgery?

17. What medical preparations do I need to make for my surgery?

18. What kind of doctor should I look for to perform my joint replacement surgery?

19. How long will I have to stay in the hospital or other health care facility for this procedure and during recovery?

APPENDIX C:

Prostate Cancer Meeting Participants

Durado Brooks, M.D.
Director of Prostate and Colorectal
Cancers
American Cancer Society
Dallas, TX

Peter Carroll, M.D.
Professor and Chair
UCSF-Mt.Zion Cancer Center
San Francisco, CA

Carolyn Clancy, M.D.
Director, Agency for Healthcare
Research and Quality
U.S. Department of Health and Human
Services
Rockville, MD

Cheryl Damberg, Ph.D.
Senior Policy Analyst
RAND
Santa Monica, CA

Jessica T. Dilorenzo
E-Communications/Initiatives Project
Leader Health Care
Corporate Benefits Delivery
General Electric
Schenectady, NY

Liisa Hiatt
Project Manager
RAND
Santa Monica, CA

Richard S. Kaplan, M.D.
Chief, Clinical Investigations Branch
National Cancer Institute
Bethesda, MD

Deborah Lubeck, Ph.D.
Research Economist
UCSF Urology Outcomes Research
Group
San Francisco, CA

Mary McCabe
Acting Director, Office of
Communications
National Cancer Institute
Bethesda, MD

Elizabeth McGlynn, Ph.D.
Associate Director, RAND Health
Santa Monica, CA

Judd Moul, M.D.
Center for Prostate Disease Research
Walter Reed Army Medical Center
Uniformed Services University of the
Health Sciences
Rockville, MD

Lewis C. Musgrove
Chairman of the Board
US-Too International
Las Vegas, NV

Dennis O'Hara
Founder, Poughkeepsie Man-to-Man
ACS support group
Poughkeepsie, NY

Arnold L. Potosky, Ph.D.
Health Services Researcher
Division of Cancer Control and
Population Sciences
National Cancer Institute
Rockville, MD

Lewis Potters, M.D.
Chief Radiation Oncologist
Memorial Sloan Kettering Cancer
Center at Mercy Medical Center
Rockville Centre, NY

Lisa Schmidt, Ph.D.
Consultant
RAND
Arlington, VA

Michael Steinberg, MD
RAND Consultant
Clinical Professor of Radiation
Oncology, UCLA
Santa Monica, CA

Leon Sun, M.D., Ph.D.
Director, CPDR National Data Base
Walter Reed Army Medical Center
Uniformed Services University of the
Health Sciences
Rockville, MD

Robert Volk, Ph.D.
Associate Professor
Baylor College of Medicine, Dept of
Family and Community Medicine
Houston, TX

APPENDIX D:

Arthritis Meeting Participants

Carolyn Clancy, M.D.
Director, Agency for Healthcare Research
and Quality
U.S. Department of Health and Human
Services
Rockville, MD

Cheryl Damberg, Ph.D.
Senior Policy Analyst
RAND
Santa Monica, CA

Liisa Hiatt
Project Manager
RAND
Santa Monica, CA

Chad Helmick
Medical Epidemiologist
Health Care and Aging Studies Branch
Division of Adult and Community Health
National Center for Chronic Disease
Prevention and Health Promotion
Centers for Disease Control and Prevention
Atlanta, GA

Nancy Lane
Professor of Medicine
Division of Rheumatology
University of California at San Francisco
San Francisco, CA

Gayle Lester
Program Director
Osteoarthritis Initiative & Diagnostic
Imaging
Musculoskeletal Diseases Branch
National Institutes of Health
Bethesda, MD

Elizabeth McGlynn, Ph.D.
Associate Director, RAND Health
RAND
Santa Monica, CA

Jaya Rao
Medical Epidemiologist
Health Care and Aging Studies Branch
Division of Adult and Community Health
National Center for Chronic Disease
Prevention and Health Promotion
Centers for Disease Control and Prevention
Atlanta, GA

Sarah Sampsell
Associate Vice President, Health Promotion
Arthritis Foundation
Washington, DC

Al Siu, M.D.
Professor/Attending Physician
Mt. Sinai School of Medicine
Department of Medicine
New York, NY

Fred Wolfe, M.D.
Arthritis Research Center Foundation
Wichita, KS

REFERENCES

Adams RJ, Smith BJ, Ruffin RE. 2001. Impact of the physician's participatory style in asthma outcomes and patient satisfaction. *Annals of Allergy, Asthma and Immunology* 86:263 - 271.

American Cancer Society, http://www.cancer.org.

American College of Cardiology and American Heart Association. November 2001. *Evaluation and Management of Chronic Heart Failure in the Adult.* American College of Cardiology/American Heart Association Guidelines.

American College of Radiology. *American College of Radiology Appropriateness Criteria—Epilepsy,* 1999.

Australian Orthopaedic Association National Joint Replacement Registry website http://www.dmac.adelaide.edu.au/aoanjrr/pt_info_August_2002.pdf.

Barry MJ. 1999. Involving patients in medical decisions: How can physicians do better? *Journal of the American Medical Association* 282:2356 - 2357.

Bates GW and Bates SR. 1996. The economics of infertility: Developing an infertility managed care plan. *American Journal of Obstetrics and Gynecology* 174 (4):1200 - 1207.

Battacharya S and Hall M. 2000. Cost-effective treatment of couples with infertility. *Lancet* 355 (9197):2.

Bellamy N, Buchanan WW, Goldsmith CH, et al. 1988. Validation study of WOMAC: A health status instrument for measuring clinically important patient relevant outcomes to antirheumatic drug therapy in patients with osteoarthritis of the hip or knee. *Journal of Rheumatology* 15:1833 - 40.

Benbadis SR and Tatum WO. 2001. Advances in the treatment of epilepsy. *American Family Physician* 64(1):91 - 98.

Benson K and Hartz AJ. 2000. A comparison of observational studies and randomized controlled trials. *New England Journal of Medicine* 342 (25):1878 - 1886.

Berland GK, Elliott MN, Morales LS, et al. 2001. Health information on the Internet: Accessibility, quality and readability in English and Spanish. *Journal of the American Medical Association* 285:2612 - 2621.

Blanchard CG, Labrecque MS, Ruckdeschel JC, et al. 1988. Information and decision-making preferences of hospitalized adult cancer patients. *Social Science and Medicine* 27:1139 - 1145.

Boberg EW, Gustafson DH, Hawkins RP, et al. 1995. Development, acceptance, and use patterns of a computer-based education and social support system for people living with AIDS/HIV infection. *Computers in Human Behavior* 11:289 - 311.

Braddock CH, Edwards KA, Hasenberg NM, et al. 1999. Informed decision-making in outpatient practice: time to get back to basics. *Journal of the American Medical Association* 282:2313 - 2320.

Brandeis J, Pashos CL, Henning JM, et al. 2000. A nationwide charge comparison of the principal treatments for early-stage prostate carcinoma. *Cancer* 89 (8):1792 - 1798.

Browne TR and Holmes, GL. 2001. Primary care: Epilepsy. *New England Journal of Medicine* 344 (15):1145 - 1151.

Centers for Disease Control and Prevention. 2001. *Arthritis: The Nation's Leading Cause of Disability*. National Center for Chronic Disease Prevention and Health Promotion, U.S. Department of Health and Human Services.

Centers for Disease Control and Prevention. 1995. *Prostate Cancer: Can we Reduce Mortality While Preserving Quality-of-life?* At-a-Glance 1994 - 1995. U.S. Department of Health and Human Services, Public Health Service.

Clancy CM, Cebul RD, Williams SV. 1988. Guiding individual decisions: A randomized, controlled trial of decision analysis. *American Journal of Medicine* 84:283 - 288.

Clark JA, Wray NP, Ashton CM. 2001. Living with treatment decisions: Regrets and quality-of-life among men treated for metastatic prostate cancer. *Journal of Clinical Oncology* 19:72 - 80.

Cooper GS. 1986. An analysis of the costs of infertility. *American Journal of Public Health* 76 (8):1018 - 1019.

Deber RB and Thompson GG. 1987. Who still prefers aggressive surgery for breast cancer? *Archives of Internal Medicine* 147:1543 - 1547.

Deber RB, Kraetschmer N, Irvine J. 1996. What role do patients wish to play in treatment decision-making? *Archives of Internal Medicine* 156:1414 - 1420.

Degner LF and Sloan JA. 1992. Decision-making during serious illness: What role do patients really want to play? *Journal of Clinical Epidemiology* 45:941 - 950.

Dunn AS, Shridharani KV, Lou W, et al. 2001. Physician-patient discussions of controversial cancer screening tests. *American Journal of Preventive Medicine* 20:130 - 134.

Easton BT. 2001. Evaluation and treatment of the patient with osteoarthritis. *Journal of Family Practice* 50 (9):791 - 802.

Edwards A and Elwyn G. 2001. Understanding risk and lessons for clinical risk communication about treatment preferences. *Quality in Health Care* 10 (Suppl I):i9 - i13.

Edwards A, Elwyn G, Gwyn R. 1999. General practice registrar responses to the use of different risk communication tools in simulated consultations: A focus group study. *British Medical Journal* 319:749 - 752.

Edwards AGK, Hood K, Matthews EJ, et al. 2000. The effectiveness of one-to-one risk communication interventions in health care: a systematic review. *Medical Decision Making* 20:290 - 297.

Epilepsy. 1996. *Vital and Health Statistics.* Series 10, No. 200.

Epilepsy Foundation of America website, http://www.efa.org.

Fox, S and Rainie L. 2000. *The Online Health Care Revolution: How the Web Helps Americans Take Better Care of Themselves.* Washington, DC, Pew Charitable Trusts.

Freund D, Lave J, Clancy C, et al. 1999. Patient outcomes research teams: contribution to outcomes and effectiveness research. *Annual Review of Public Health* 20:337 - 359.

Fries JF. 1976. A data bank for the clinician? *New England Journal of Medicine* 294:1400 - 1402.

Frosch DL and Kaplan RM. 1999. Shared decision-making in clinical medicine: Past research and future directions. *American Journal of Preventive Medicine* 17:285 - 294.

Frosch DL, Kaplan RM, Felitti V. 2001. Evaluation of two methods to facilitate shared decision-making for men considering the prostate-specific antigen test. *Journal of General Internal Medicine* 16:391 - 398.

Gattellari M, Butow PN, Tattersall MHN. 2001. Sharing decisions in cancer care. *Social Science and Medicine* 52:1865 - 1878.

Goel V, Sawka CA, Thiel EC, Gort EH, O'Connor AM. 2001. Randomized trial of a patient decision aid for choice of surgical treatment for breast cancer. *Medical Decision Making* 21(1): 1-6.

Gomberg-Maitland M, Baran DA, Fuster V. February 2001. Treatment of congestive heart failure: guidelines for the primary care physician and the heart failure specialist, *Archives of Internal Medicine* 161(3):342 - 352.

Guadagnoli E and Ward P. 1998. Patient participation in decision-making. *Social Science and Medicine* 47:329 - 339.

Gustafson DH, McTavish F, Pingree S, et al. 1996. *Final Report: Feasibility Study to Assess Impact of Computer-Based Support for Medicare Eligible Women with Breast Cancer.* Final Report to the Health Care Financing Administration. U.S. Department of Health and Human Services.

Hersey JC, Matheson J, Lohr KN. 1997. *Consumer Health Informatics And Patient Decision-Making: Final Report.* AHCPR Publication No. 98-N001.

Hibbard JH, Slovic P, Peters E, Finucane ML. 2002. Strategies for reporting health plan performance information to consumers: Evidence from controlled studies. *Health Services Research* 37:291 - 313.

Hibbard JH, Slovic P, Jewett JJ. 1997. Informing consumer decisions in health care: Implications from decision-making research. *Milbank Quarterly* 75:395 - 414.

Hing MMS, Laupacis A, O'Connor AM, et al. 2000. Development of a decision aid for patients with atrial fibrillation who are considering antithrombotic therapy. *Journal of General Internal Medicine* 15:723 - 730.

Hlatky MA, Lee KL, Harrell FE, Jr., et al. 1984. Tying clinical research to patient care by use of an observational data base. *Statistics in Medicine* 3:375 - 384.

Holmberg L, Bill-Axelson A, Helgesen R, et al. 2002. A randomized trial comparing radical prostatectomy with watchful waiting in early prostate cancer. *New England Journal of Medicine* 347:781 - 789.

Jemal A, Thomas A, Murray T, et al. 2002. Cancer statistics, 2002. *California Cancer Journal Clin* 52:23 - 47.

Jones R, Pearson J, McGregor S, et al. 1999. Randomized trial of personalized computer based information for cancer patients. *British Medical Journal* 319:1241 - 1247.

Kamas G. 1995. A pilot evaluation of an informatics tool for patients with lower back pain. FHP HealthCare, Unpublished manuscript.

Kennelly C and Bowling A. 2001. Suffering in deference: A focus group study of older cardiac patients' preferences for treatment and perception of risk. *Quality in Health Care* 10 (Suppl. I):i23 - i28.

Koller WC. Fall 1993. Epidemiology of Parkinson's disease, *World Parkinson's Disease Association Newsletter*.

Legorreta AP, Brooks RJ, Leibowitz AN, et al. 1996. Cost of breast cancer treatment: A 4-year longitudinal study. *Archives of Internal Medicine* 156 (19):2197 - 2201.

Li TCM, Sherman H, Cook EF, et al. 1984. The selective impact of a cardiology data bank on physicians' therapeutic recommendations. *Medical Decision Making* 4(2):165 - 176.

Litwin MS, Steinberg M, Malin J, et al. 2000. *Prostate Cancer Patient Outcomes and Choice of Providers: Development of an Infrastructure for Quality Assessment*. RAND. Santa Monica, CA MR-1227-BF.

Lloyd AJ. 2001. The extent of patients' understanding of the risk of treatments. *Quality in Health Care* 10(Suppl I):i14 - i18.

Man-Son-Hing M, Laupacis A, O'Connor AM, et al. 1999. A patient decision aid regarding antithrombotic therapy for stroke prevention in atrial fibrillation: A randomized controlled trial. *Journal of the American Medical Association* 282:737 - 743.

Mantel N. 1983. Cautions on the use of medical data bases. *Statistics in Medicine* 2:355 - 362.

McKinstry B. 2000. Do patients wish to be involved in decision-making in the consultation? A cross sectional survey with video vignettes. *British Medical Journal* 321:867 - 871.

McPherson K, Britton AR, Wennberg JE. 1997. Are randomized controlled trials controlled? Patient preferences and unblind trials. *Journal of the Royal Society of Medicine* 90: 652 - 656.

Morbidity and Mortality Weekly Report. 1994. *Current Trends Prevalence of Self-Reported Epilepsy—United States, 1986-1990.* Centers for Disease Prevention and Control, US Department of Health and Human Services. 43(44); 810 - 814.

Montgomery AA, Fahey T, Peters TJ, et al. 2000. Evaluation of computer based clinical decision support system and risk chart for management of hypertension in primary care: Randomized controlled trial. *British Medical Journal* 320:686 - 690.

Mosher WD, Bachrach CA. 1996. Understanding US fertility: Continuity and change in the national survey of family growth, 1988-1995. *Family Planning Perspectives* 28(1): 4 - 12.

Murray E, Davis H, Tai SS, et al. 2001a. Randomized controlled trial of an interactive multimedia decision aid on hormone replacement therapy in primary care. *British Medical Journal* 323:490 - 493.

Murray E, Davis H, Tai SS, et al. 2001b. Randomized controlled trial of an interactive multimedia decision aid on benign prostatic hypertrophy in primary care. *British Medical Journal* 323:493 - 496.

National Comprehensive Cancer Network. *2000/2001 Breast Cancer Guidelines.* http://www.nccn.com/physicanfls/index.html.

National Institutes of Health. *Breast Cancer Fact Sheet 2001.* http://cra.nci.nih.gov/3_types_cancer/breast_cancer.htm.

National Heart, Lung, and Blood Institute. 1996. *Congestive Heart Failure in the United States: A New Epidemic. Data Fact Sheet.* National Institutes of Health.

National Multiple Sclerosis Society. 2001. *The Multiple Sclerosis Information Sourcebook.* http://www.national/mssociety.org/sourcebook.asp.

O'Connor AM, Stacey D, Rovner D, et al. 2003. Decision aids for people facing health treatment or screening decisions (Cochrane Review). In: The Cochrane Library, Issue 1. Oxford: Update Software.

O'Connor AM, Fiset V, DeGrasse C, et al. 1999. Decision aids for patients considering options affecting cancer outcomes: Evidence of efficacy and policy implications. *Journal of the National Cancer Institute Monographs* 25:67 - 80.

Parkinson's Action Network. 1999. *The Cost of Parkinson's Disease.* http://www.parkinsonsaction.org.

Partin AW, Kattan MW, Subong ENP, et al. 1997. Combination of prostate-specific antigen, clinical stage and Gleason score to predict pathological stage of localized prostate cancer: A multi-institutional update. *Journal of the American Medical Association* 277(18):1445 - 1451.

Peto R and Baigent C. 1998. Trials: The next 50 years. *British Medical Journal* 317:1170 - 1171.

Pienta KJ, Sandler H, Sanda MG, Hollenbeck BK, eds. 2001. Prostate Cancer. In: *Cancer Management: A Multidisciplinary Approach,* Pazdur R, Cola L, Hoskins WJ, Wagman LD, eds., Melville, NY: PRR, Inc.

Polman CH and Uitdehaag BMJ. 2000. Drug treatment of multiple sclerosis, *British Medical Journal* 321:490 - 494.

Pound CR, Partin AW, Epstein JI, et al. 1997. Outcomes following anatomical radical retropubic prostatectomy: Patterns of recurrence and cancer control. *Urology Clinics of North America* 24:395 - 406.

Robinson A and Thomson R. 2001. Variability in patient preferences for participating in medical decision-making: Implications for the use of decision support tools. *Quality in Health Care* 10 (Suppl. I): i34 - i38.

Slovic P. 1995. The construction of preference. *American Psychologist* 50:364 - 371.

Sommers SD and Ramsey SD. 1999. A review of quality-of-life evaluations in prostate cancer. *Pharmacoeconomics* 16(2):127 - 140.

Stephen EH and Chandra A. 2000. Use of infertility services in the United States: 1995. *Family Planning Perspectives* 32 (3):132 - 137.

Stevenson FA, Barry CA, Britten N, et al. 2000. Doctor-patient communication about drugs: The evidence for shared decision making. *Social Science and Medicine* 50:829 - 840.

Strull WM, Lo B, Charles G. 1984. Do patients want to participate in medical decision making? *Journal of the American Medical Association* 252:2990 - 2994.

Tversky A and Kahneman D. 1981. The framing of decisions and the psychology of choice. *Science* 211:453 - 458.

Vaiana ME and McGlynn EA. 2002. What cognitive science tells us about the design of reports for consumers. *Medical Care Research and Review* 59:3 - 35.

Vertinsky IB, Thompson WA, Uyeno D. 1974. Measuring consumer desire for participation in clinical decision-making. *Health Services Research* 9:121 - 133.

Volk RJ, Cass AR, Spann SJ. 1999. A randomized controlled trial of shared decision-making for prostate cancer screening. *Archives of Family Medicine* 8:333 - 340.

Wagner EH, Barrett P, Barry MJ, et al. 1995. The effect of a shared decision-making program on rates of surgery for benign prostatic hyperplasia: Pilot results. *Medical Care* 33:765 - 770.

Watt S. 2000. Clinical decision-making in the context of chronic illness. *Health Expectations* 3:6 - 16.

Wennberg JE, Barry MJ, Fowler FJ, et al. 1993. Outcomes research, PORTs, and health care reform. *Annals of the New York Academy of Sciences* 703: 52 - 62.

Whetten-Goldstein K, Sloan FA, Goldstein LB, et al. 1998. A comprehensive assessment of the cost of multiple sclerosis in the United States. *Multiple Sclerosis* 4(3):419 - 425.

Young R. 1999. Update on Parkinson's disease. *American Family Physician* 59(8):2155 - 2170.